Tribute
To The
Black Woman

Written By
M.P.E.R.O.R.

Edited By
Mylia Tiye Mal Jaza

Tribute
To The
Black Woman

Written By
M.P.E.R.O.R.

Edited By
Mylia Tiye Mal Jaza

Cover Art By
Inkosi Design Studio
Kevin Bryant

Self-Publishing Associate
The Conglomerate – Be Published
Mari "Mary" Jefferson

Tribute To The Black Woman
Copyright © 2007 M.P.E.R.O.R.

All Rights Reserved.

Publisher Contact Information:

BePublished.Org
P.O. Box 8324
Jackson, MS 39284
www.bepublished.biz
mari@bepublished.org
(972) 880-8316

Author Contact Information:

M.P.E.R.O.R.
mperor.com
mperor.7p.com
myspace.com/mperor01
myspace.com/mperor25
mperor7@hotmail.com
mperor@excite.com
(636) 447-3634

ISBN: 978-0-6151-6332-1

Printed in the United States of America

First Edition

Table of Contents

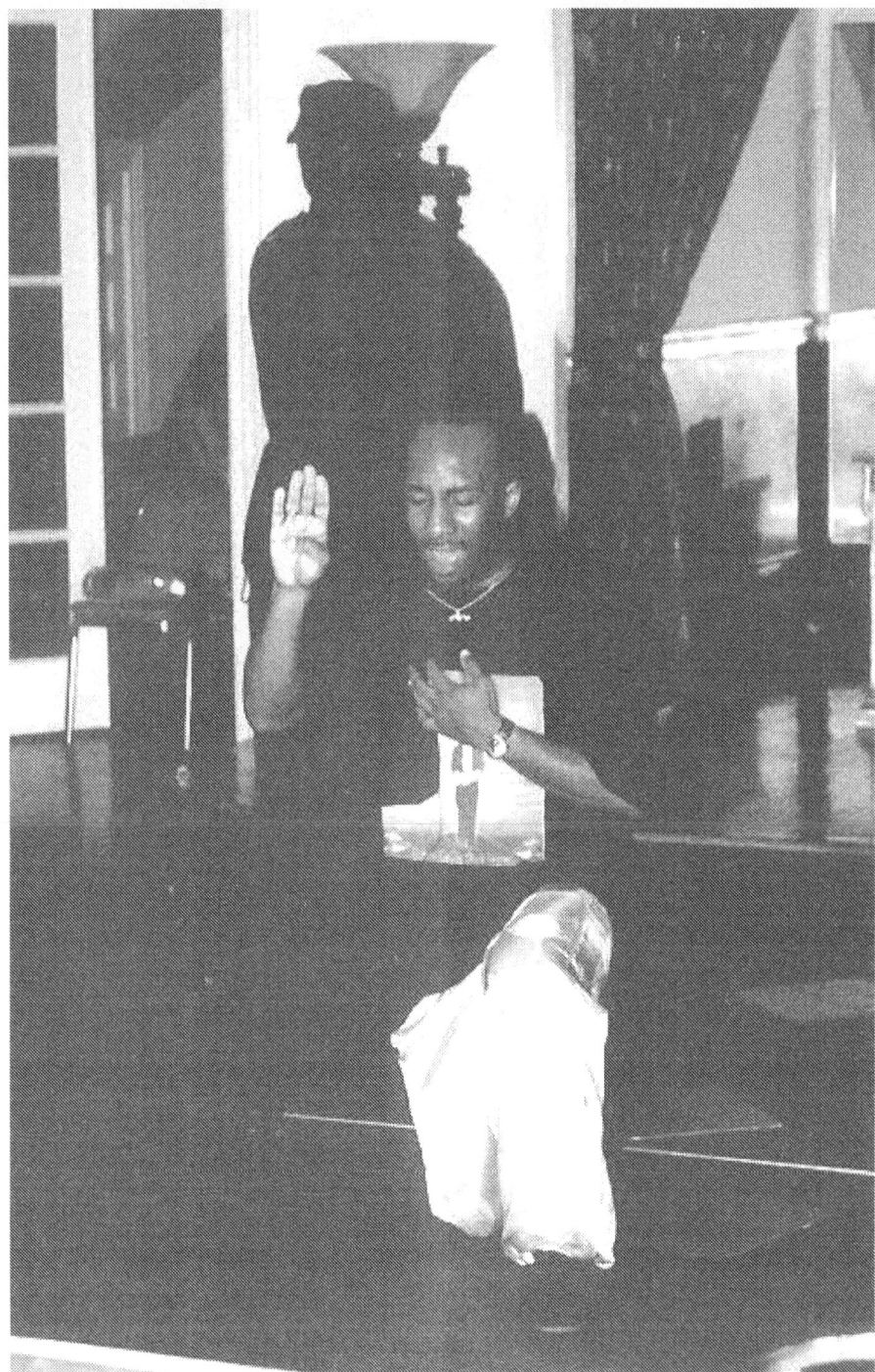

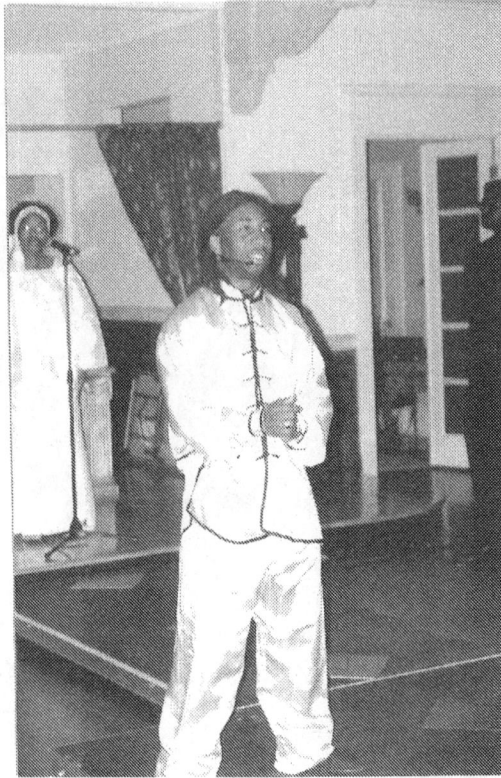

Extra spiritual special thanks to
Mary "Goddess Sage" Jefferson

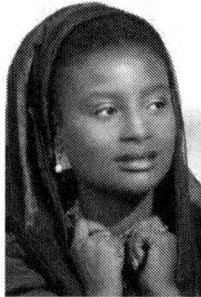

I and i thank you with mind, heart and soul. Just as Christ was born during a crisis, during my crisis, you helped me borne the Christ of this book.

"No revolution has been won without discipline."
– Che Guevara

Acknowledgements

Give thanks and praises to THE MOST HIGH. I must thank THE MOST HIGH for OUR ANCESTORS because if they would not have Been, then we would not Be.

Peace to my Earthly parents, Queen Mother Edith Holmes and King Father Lee Holmes Sr. Peace also to my other family members.

Much Respect to the Royal Entourage, A.B.T. (All Brothuz Together), Panther Protection, F.O.I. (Fruit of Islam), R.E.A.L. (Reality Expected And Lived), Protective Services, and all who are about turning gangsters into guerillas. Long Live!

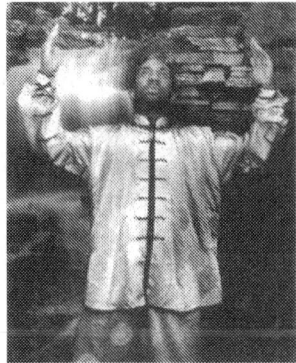

Guerilla love to: Keith Minor, Greg Walker, Nelson, Ringo, Darrell Cobbs, James "Br. J." Ray, the Merchant family, Yoel, Nijah Kamau, Tizir "Min. Truth" Smith, Roderick "The Seeker" Reed, Raynard Shelton, Man of War a.k.a. Meru, Chango, Rahotep "O," James "Lord J4" Muhammad, Dragon, Larry "Tehuti" Edwards, Brown "Sleeping Giant," Ronald Muhammed, World's Champion trainer Master Ron Smith, Br. Paul, Br. Malik, Br. Elton, Br. Adoni, and Charles Cuttery. To everyone who has supported me, you are not forgotten. Never forget!

Much love to Cathryn Blue, Wrath of G.O.D.

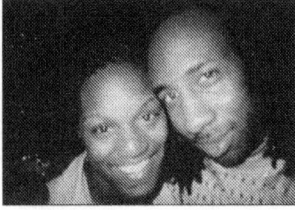

Innertainment, T.R.U.T.H. Squad, Osiris, Chakrush, Elixer, Ra "The Masta" Armageddon a.k.a. Braides, Thunder, Black Onyx, Erica McDaniels, Oneness, Yonasda Lonewolf, Cappadonna and RZA of Wu-Tang, Warrior Woman, Latecia Favors, the Hebrew Israelite Community, Samantha Raheem, Ashra Kwesi Dr. Ben, John Henrik Clarke (Peace Be Unto Him), Yahkhanah, and Dr. York and the Nuwaupian Nation (Ancient Egiptian Order).

One love to Falaq, Mea Epps, M.K. Stallings, Divine Tea (sistakeeper.com), Mocha, Poetry in Motion, Floyd Boykin Jr. a.k.a.

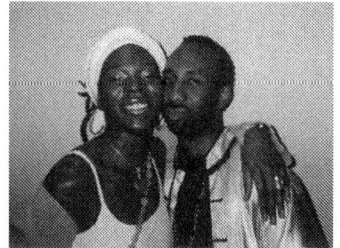

Impakt, Chill, Amina, Ancient Newcomer, Black On Black Rhyme, Blackberry, India.Arie, Leah Love, Anthony Stewart (videographer), Black Reign, First World, Ujamaa, Knowing Books & Café, ONE Love, Golden Grocer, Eternity, Shang,

Vintage Vinyl, R.O.A.R. (Rage of All Righteousness), Fresh Voice (we gotta do something together), Kanita "Emoetry" Hillard (thanks for taking care of me in Houston), Sun Star

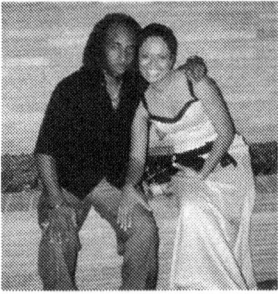

Divine, Sally's World (you have some hot creations), All Stars (I see you Black), Big Ant, Brother Alvin, Jacque Land & Leata Price (Platinum Group), Professor Griff of Public Enemy, Pastor Ray Hagins of African Village, Tony and Patricia Simms at Bread Box Studios (when you drink water, remember its source), Khalif Amen Ra, Mark Spielberg, Soultide, Alter States of Consciousness, Dr. Afua - my personal acupuncturist and my loctitian, Karen "Red Dred" Martin, Dubtronics, Yard Squad, Inkosi (Kevin Bryant,

thanks for the support from day one), Kevin Johnson Post-Dispatch (good looking out), Bits & Pieces (Katt & Jia, one!), Holiday, Ms. Nterpretation, Teke, Steve "God Man" Ward, Fly DX

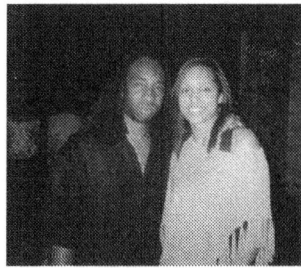

(KRS-One of St. Louis, Brotha, you are hip-hop in St. Louis), Flex (right on for the hip-hop kalostenics), Rachael Williams, Laron Epps, Jeanetta Wilkerson, my Muay Thai Family, Fuji,

Black Lion Productions, Rikkathon, Ajumma Muhammed, and Anthony Shyheed (thanks for having my back. Guerilla love).

Also, thanks and love to: Universal Afrikan Peoples Organization, Better Family Life, National Black United Front, St. Louis Black Rep, St. Louis American, St. Louis Argus, I & i Gallery, India Palace, Pharoah Gerumba (The World's Greatest Artist), K.G. Harris & Assoc., Déjà Vu radio

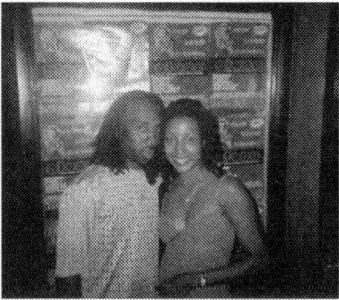

personality (Sistah, even though we haven't met, I and i thank you for your support), Queen Isis Jones (thanks for looking out in New Orleans and "Being." Guerilla love), Kevy Kev (right on for stepping up on my behalf. Long Live!), D.J. Needles (continue to "Be"), D.J. Knock Knock (I hear you knocking, God), JM3 DJs, D.J. Jess Trip'n, D.J. Quinn, and the Council of Elders — Duane McGowan, Quadir, Oman, and James Henderson.

Special expressions of gratitude and replenishment are greatly extended to my lifelong guide, my Earthly and spiritual brother, Jermaine "Bam Bam" Andre' aka "The Product." Keep up all you do to protect our women and teach them to protect themselves through AWSD - Andre's

Women's Street Defense (andresmmaacademy.com). You are far more than the World Fighting Alliance No Holds Bar World Champion and four-time U.S. Kickboxing champion! Your teaching women of all ages self-defense tactics through safe, easy and fun seminars, manuals and videos continues to motivate me to create new ways to help our women help themselves as well. Thank you for allowing me opportunities to get involved. And, please accept from me a portion of proceeds from the *Tribute To The Black Woman* CD and book to benefit your Women's Street Defense fund.

To all of you who haven't been named, please know you and your contributions and support over the years were not in vain and have not been forgotten. I offer many praises to JAH for all you have done to show me the nurturing support throughout the years. I pray I may be as much of a benefit to your spirit and life's work as you have been to mine.

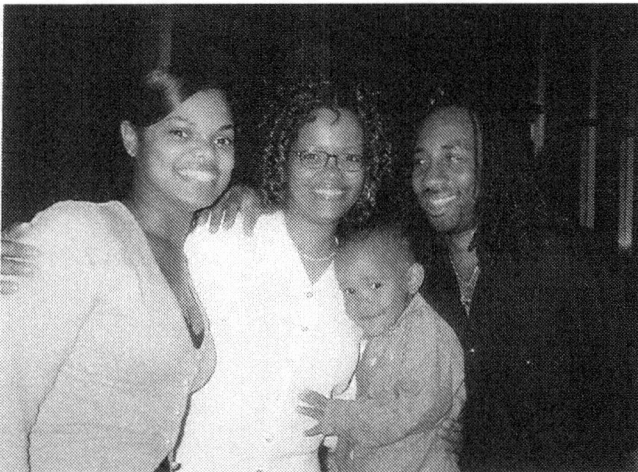

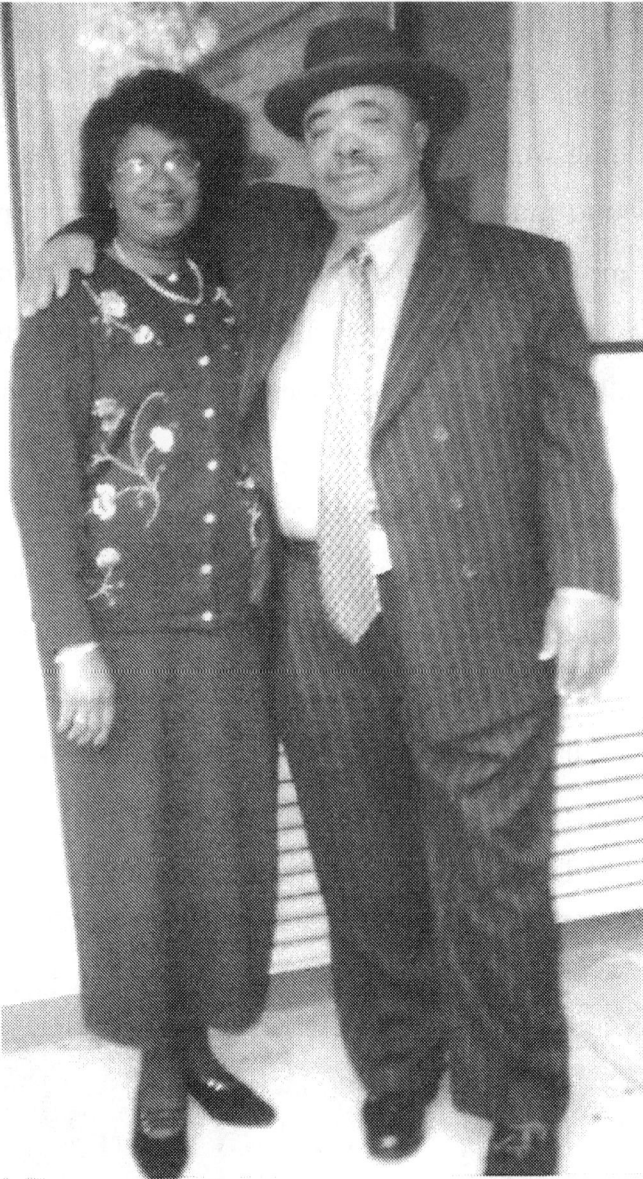

Queen Mother and King Father
who birthed and nurtured M.P.E.R.O.R.

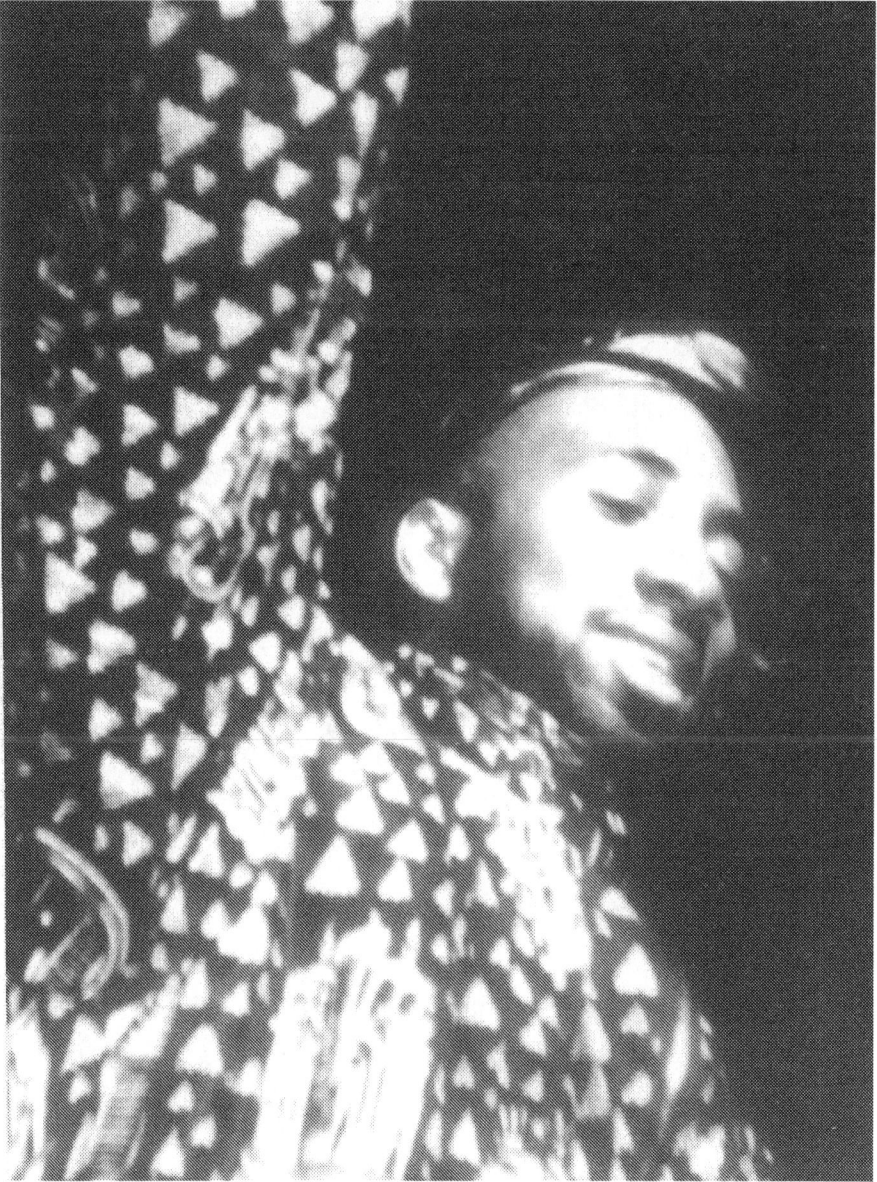

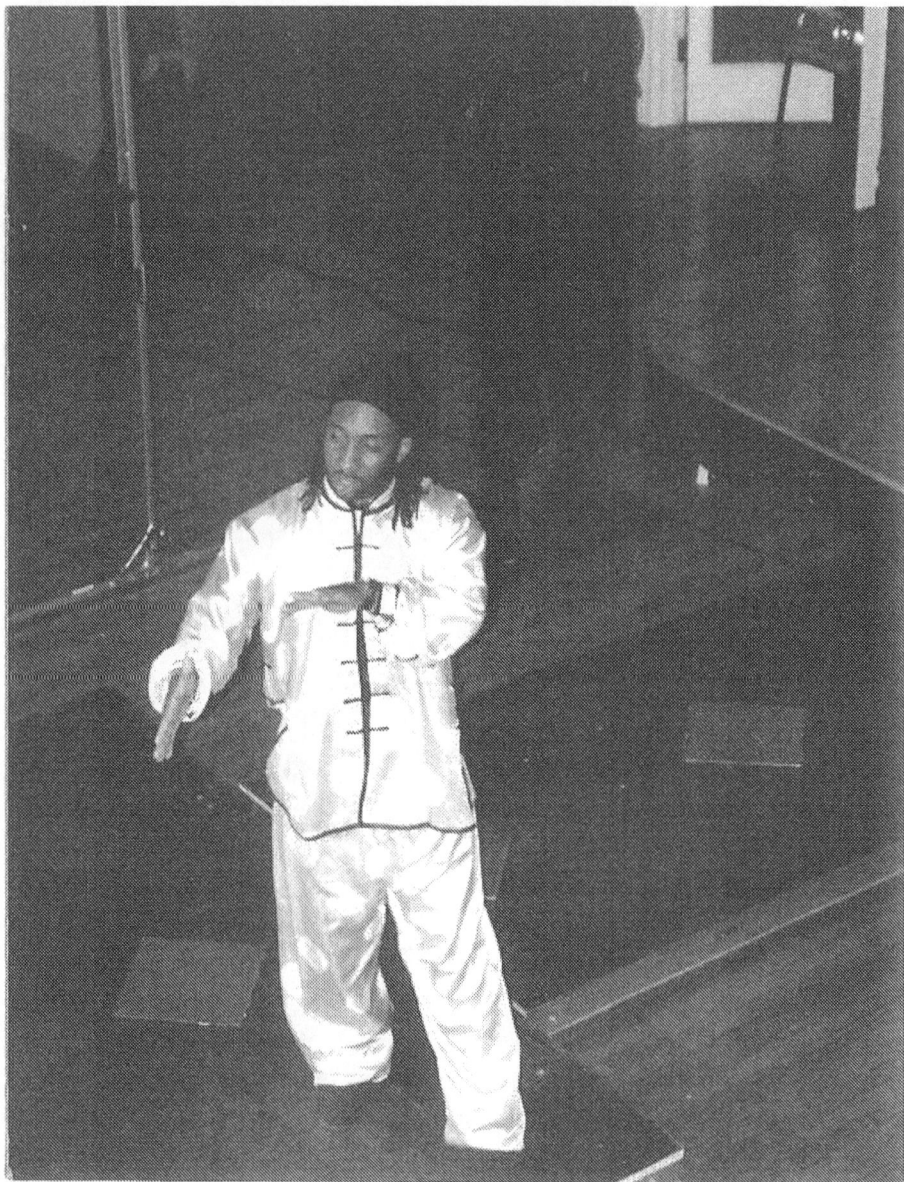

Ntrodukshun

Tribute To The Black Woman has been inspired by relationships I have had with Black women such as my grandmothers, Queen Mother, aunts, cousins, friends, and, of course, women I have been involved with on that other level.

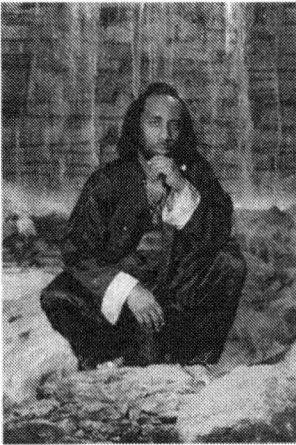

Instead of taking the most common (i.e., negative) attitude when things don't go according to plans in a relationship, I began to follow the uncharted path. I started asking questions like: "Why are Black women hurt and angry? Why do Black men seem to go ridiculously overboard in disrespecting Black women? And, why have Black women started accepting Black men who go ridiculously overboard in disrespecting them?"

The self-realization I have come to is: We Are Phukked Up, <u>And</u> More Than We Could Ever Imagine. This is apparent any time you are listening to music with words which constantly speak of you not being shit, and watch movies and read magazines which reflect you not being shit. Brought up in school systems as well as a social society which clearly says you ain't shit, it's unfortunate that our only response is that of a pig squirming in mud. The filthier the pig gets, the more the pig squeals and squirms in its enjoyment.

How in Hell (literally) can the masses of Black women appreciate *Tribute To The Black Woman* when the masses of Black women have accepted "Fuck You Bitch" as their mantra? Even subconsciously, it has been accepted when you don't support or know how to appreciate a brotha who gives respect to such greatness (You, Black Woman).

No other genre of music degrades, disrespects, and exploits a culture's women more than hip-hop and rap. There are some very beautiful Jewish women, for example. Jews control this entire music, movie, magazine, and entertainment industry. As beautiful as Jewish women are, why aren't their men letting them drop it like it's hot? Their women tend to be in positions like public relations, management, etc. This is how they employ "their" women.

The reality is that we all have issues. Our (Black people's) issues are more tragic and traumatizing than any other people's on planet Earth.

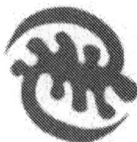

Once there was a boy child walking in the mountains. The child found a fallen hawk's nest. He took an egg from the fallen hawk's nest and brought it to the farm where the child lived. The child put the egg in the chicken coup. A hen sat on the egg and when the egg hatched, a hawk came out.

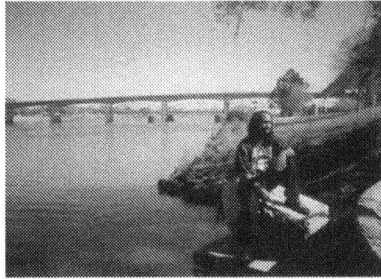

One day, the hawk was playing with the chickens and some hawks flew overhead. Well, the hawk said, "Those birds look like me. I want to fly too." The chickens looked at the hawk and said, "You can't fly. You're just a chicken."

The hawk was born and raised in Compton (naw, just kidding) as a chicken. This was all the hawk knew: the life of a chicken. Although the life of the chicken was all the hawk knew, the hawk felt greater than a chicken inside.

One day, the hawk was with himself, thinking of the negative things the chickens told him. While the hawk was thinking of these things, some more hawks flew over his head. The hawk just erased all the negativity it was taught, took off running, spread his wings and was flying with the other hawks.

When the hawk flew over the chickens who said, "You can't fly. You're just a chicken," the hawk saw that those chickens were hawks too.

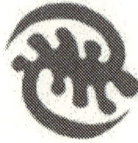

God created the Black man and Black woman. From God's Creation, the White man made Niggers, Niggas and Niggaz. No matter how you spell it, it identifies you as a product of the White man.

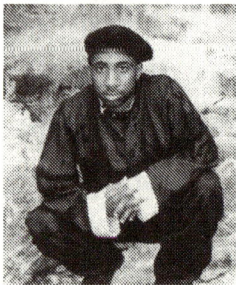

People, I and i* spread my wings by spreading what little wisdom I have to educate as many people as possible. If all we think we are is niggas, bitches, and thugs (chickens), then those are all we will ever be – no matter how much money you have. Because, if you give a slave money, all you have is a slave who thinks he's now rich. I and i have come forth to show and prove that we (Black people) are Mothers and Fathers of civilizations, Queens and Kings of the planet Earth, and Goddesses and Gods of the universe.

I and i pray that *Tribute To The Black Woman* will help re-establish the trust and love which I feel is gone between the Black Man and Black Woman.

"There is no one higher than your child.

There is nothing greater than yourself."

– Dr. Ben (Respect to the Grand Lodge of Wa'at).

The sacred teaching of OUR ANCESTORS says, "You can respect and not love, but you can't love and not respect."

TRUE GUIDANCE

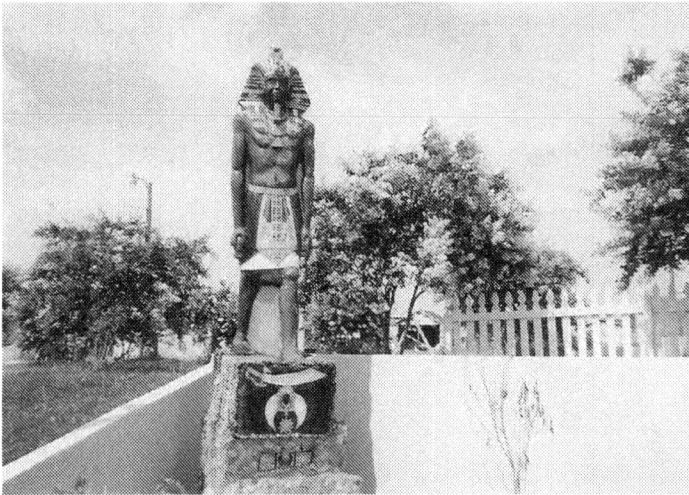

* I and i: "I" represents the CREATOR. "i" represents myself.

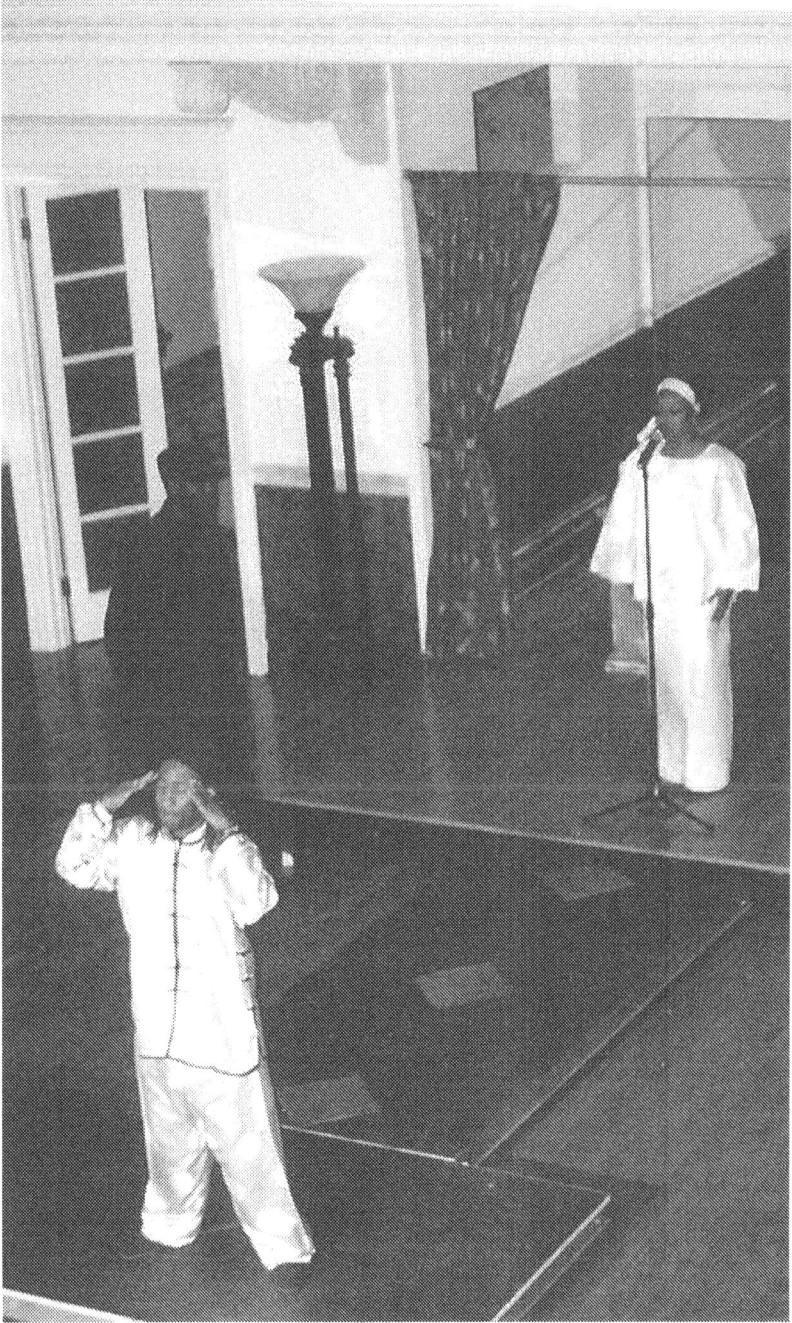

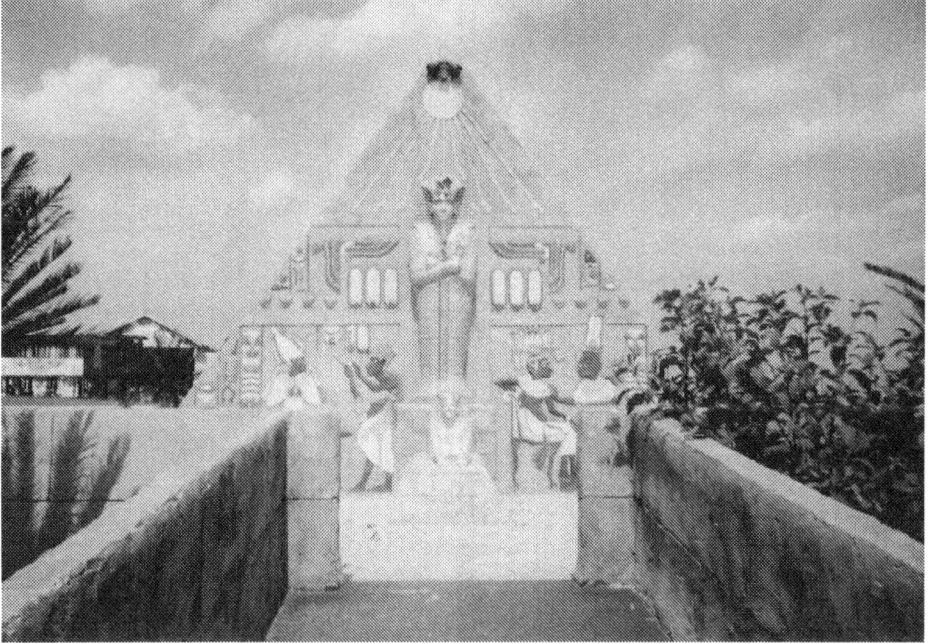

Know Thy Self

In many of the sacred tombs and temples in ancient Africa, "Know Thy Self" were the primary words written on the walls. In many of our sacred holy books – such as the Bible, Koran, Metu Neter, Sanskrit, etc. – "Know Thy Self" is written.

OUR ANCESTORS knew that once we were able to identify ourselves as the "one life that dwells as the self in all beings,"* we would be able to reach our greatest potential. There is an Egyptian proverb which says "For one to search for their soul in the world is an illusion." So, many of us look outside of ourselves for the greatness in ourselves, including me.

Blessed Be!

Deception occurs when you are divided,
Truth appears when you are whole.
Uniting male and female brings illumination,
The real master is a perfect light.

No one is ineligible to know higher truth. When concentration, energy, and thinking are scattered, we cannot break out of ignorance. The diversity and contradictions of existence confuse us, and appearances deceive us.

Q: Do we need a master to help us in the struggle to know the truth?

A: In the beginning we do. What is not often said is that the human master is but a temporary and imperfect manifestation of the ultimate truth. Without a master, you cannot make a beginning.

If you never look beyond the person, you will never attain the entirety. A good master leads you to the true master within. Only that master, who is your own higher self, can adequately answer all questions.

Once you unite all elements within yourself, metaphorically referred to as the uniting of male and female, the light that dispels darkness appears. Just as all colored light together makes colorless light, so too does the combination of all our facets result in the integration of our polarities. When this happens, you will "see" a light in your meditations. This light brings knowledge. That is why it is called the true master.**

* This quote comes from Metu Neter, Vol. 2.
**This passage taken from 365 TAO.

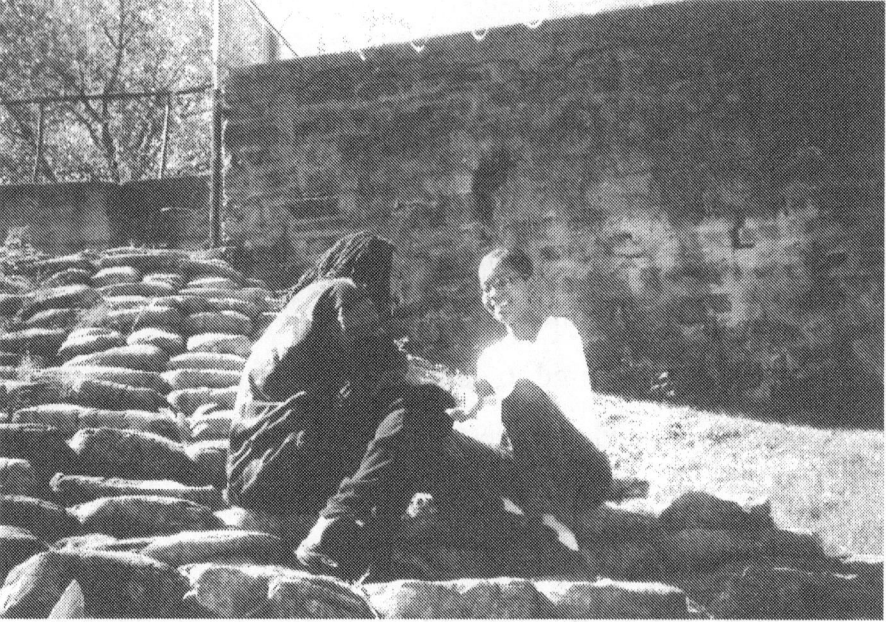

Mental Loving

"There's nothing physical about it. It's all in the mental."

- Professor X of X-Clan, PBUH.*

Mental loving is a lesson which focuses on learning to love the mental and celebrating that love in the physical.

Let's be real, peeps. Most of us please ourselves mentally more than anyone else ever could. So, to have someone spark your brain cell and ignite a fusion which brings light in any dark confusion can be quite fulfilling.

If we go with the basis of "out of darkness comes light" (Genesis), we should know that it will never be so dark in our lives that we won't be able to bring light out of that darkness.

TRUE GUIDANCE

*PBUH — Peace Be Upon Him.

Mental Loving

Many brothuz claim to represent the righteous,

I still choose to live righteous despite this.

I'm too old to be a player with origin of a mack,

Now, I'm back in black

Standing in square right and xzact.

My ways and actions show and prove

What I'm made of.

My mother has the tender love;

My father has the tough love.

When tender and tough come together,

It's intended

To bring forth and protect justice

When it's offended.

You are the justice I must protect

With my life, my blood, my tears,

but most of all my sweat.

The more we sweat together,

The less we have to bleed.

Our wants and needs become one

The day I plant the seed.

When the mental iz pure the soul iz pure.

A spiritual connection,

This iz an immaculate conception.

Just like Buddah.

Just like Krishna.

Just like Yeshua

Who you know as Jesus.

You are the moon of my reflection.

I'm the sun

In the center of the universe

Spreading rays of mental loving.

A man has the X and Y chromosomes,

A woman only has an X

And turns a house into a home.

A woman iz stronger, as a man I have no shame,

Cuz women can deal with more emotional pain.

One thing that really impressed me about you,

Iz you don't like to wear them damn Daizy Dukes.

Either Sistahs don't love themselves

Or they just don't care,

Cuz I see sistahs in them shorts

Daizy Duke wouldn't even wear.

Sistahs like that can't fade a brotha like me.

They let their body do the talking

Cuz they're struggling mentally.

Sex iz divine but now it's become a hobby,

Too many people have separated

Their mind from their body.

We must raise our conscious

To anoint a mental resurrection.

This iz my way of showing you affection.

There's nothing physical about it —

It's all in the mental.

Wizdom iz an orgasm glorifying the holy temple.

Mentally caressing you, mentally rubbing

Your temple down with a little mental loving.

Since the Greeks defined love,

There's been a mess here since.

So don't look at this as a date but an xperience.

We come together to xplore each others mental.

Xploring the physical iz too common and so simple.

Time destroys all things — time could never be late.

We can stop time, Queen, when we meditate.

Flesh to Flesh later comes kissing and hugging.

But for now, let's make beautiful musik

Together from our mental loving.

Unfortunately,

People tend to respond to words,

Instead of responding to reality.

Reality is, when you use the words,

"Fall in love,"

You usually get hurt

Or you break something.

We need to learn to grow in love.

Then, we will be able to rise

To love together.

TRUE GUIDANCE

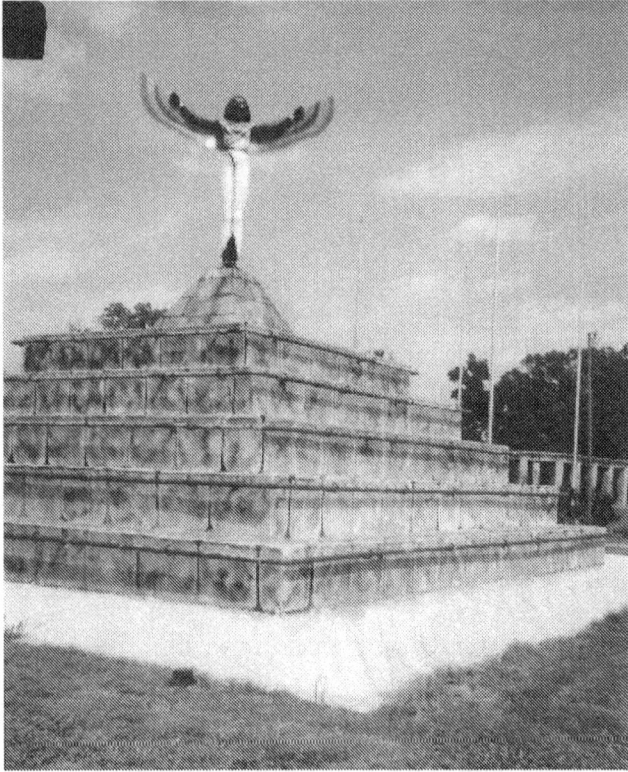

Spiritual Healing

"There is no way you can go into a wrong situation
and expect a right outcome."

- Tizir "Mr. Truth" Smith

So many relationships are doomed from the start. Have you ever looked at a couple and thought, "You know they shouldn't be together?" Let's be clear. Having these thoughts does not make you a hater, only hater proof.

There is an ancient Afrikan saying, "My inner being is too important to be held ransom to factors outside of my control."*

How many of us truly have inner peace? We have been physically assaulted, emotionally assaulted, spiritually assaulted, and psychologically assaulted for 400 plus years. We are still under this assault, no matter how sophisticated and modernized it has become. Freedom to do what you want is bondage. Freedom to do what you need to do is true freedom.**

We need spiritual healing. We want sexual healing. Unfortunately, many of us have yet to realize that our "sexual energy is our driving force for accomplishing all our goals in life. Misunderstand or misuse it and you will have no say so when it comes back and avenges you." (Metu Neter, Vol.1)

The point of all this is that we complain about situations and circumstances that we have put ourselves into because we have not been taught the importance of our sexual energy since before we were free people who became enslaved.

* This quote comes from Metu Neter, Vol. 2 Amen Truism.
**This quote comes from the book *I Am That.*

Spiritual Healing

Peace Queen Wizdom Asiatic —

I didn't come for static.

I'm stepping to you with the mathematics.

You are the zero and I am number one.

When I'm just beginning,

You have already begun

To peep my smitty and game recognize game.

But Queen, I'm not ashamed to tell you

I don't have no game.

I'm straight up on the real —

I deal with the deal.

See, hear, and feel my spiritual appeal.

I seen you from a distance

Sitting at a juice bar.

My third eye seen your reflection

From the sun, moon and star.

Now, you here Queen, and I got that feeling

That while you're chilling,

You need some spiritual healing.

A House N-I-G-G-A is what you deal with,

Who drinks and smokes weed all day.

You need to kill this.

I'm a G-O-D body

Who spreads his wisdom with everybody.

It seems you're lonely, Goddess;

You need a God in yo life.

Them Mortals ain't loving you right.

A dog thinks with his penis;

A god thinks with his mind.

The sun and moon need one another

For both of them to shine.

You may want a righteous man,

But not all the way right.

So you ended up wit a thug in yo life.

His momma couldn't raise him.

What makes you think you can?

Perhaps God's decision for you

Isn't in your plan.

A foolish woman justifies ignorance.

A prideful woman won't seek deliverance.

A strong, humble woman is a precious jewel.

She learned from a fool not to be a fool.

I'm a messenger of Ra who's always building

Bridges ova troubled waters for God's children.

At the Million Man March, I was one and a million;

But we still need spiritual healing.

Yo, Queen,

Don't think I'm into breaking up Black families.

Our families are already broken, no jokin'.

A nation can rise no higher than its woman,

But it has to be a good man and a good woman.

Sex, Salt and Peppa tried to talk about.

What you put in sex is what you get out.

The Acts of Creation are beyond a stimulation.

That's why aggravation and frustration

Rules the nation.

Our sexual drive is geared toward our life force.

If we misuse it, we get off of our life's course.

That's why they use sex to sell some of everything.

Sex has become a marketing scheme.

They have us living in our lower self-unconscious.

They tricked us wit toys; men are still boys.

Be conscious and rize up to your higher self.

When things are out of bounds,

I call penalties like a ref.

A chef serving food for thought in the struggle.

My spirit is more powerful than my muscle.

Let him run the streets

With his thugz and keep cheating.

Grab yo kids and come to the teaching.

I'm speaking and reaching everyday and weekend.

Hypocrites and heathens get spiritual beatings.

The blind start seeing;

Non-believers start believing.

In the true and living manifestation

Of my Creation,

At the end of patience is heaven. I'm blessing

My sistah and bretheren with I and i's lesson.

Words of wisdom are fulfilling

A Peace of Mind comes from Spiritual Healing.

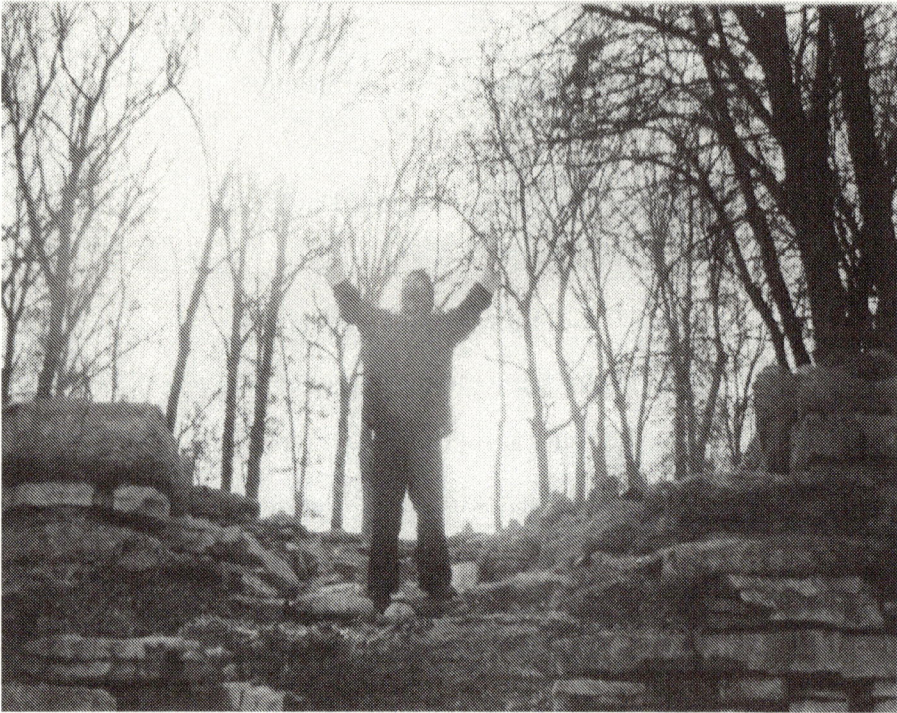

Peace of Mind

Once upon a time, I was going through a very bad break-up. It was the first time I'd ever felt love and I thought it was the end of the world.

I mean, I was on the love diet . . . losing weight because I couldn't eat. I wasn't taking baths or showers. I couldn't sleep. Just straight up trippin'. Going through withdrawals. Thinking "I ain't gon call." Then, I call. Stalking her. Just crazy shit. Started going to AA meetings and didn't even drink at the time. Going to NA meetings and wasn't a drug user. The reality was that I was in recovery cuz I was in love.

Well, one day, I and my earthly father were building (talking). I asked him, "When you become an ancestor, if you could only leave me one thing, what would it be?" My father is really into nature. He loves gardening and working outside. He loves raising, breeding, and training horses – Tennessee Walkers in particular. He's had a couple of champion show horses. I just knew when I asked him that question he was going to say something about those horses. To my surprise, he answered, "If I could only leave you one thing when I die, I would leave you a peace of mind."

Peace of Mind

As I give thanks and praises

To the MOST HIGH,

I would like to thank the MOST HIGH

for OUR ANCESTORS.

If they would not have been,

Then we would not be.

I want everyone to fasten their spiritual seatbelts.

We're about to take a ride through the cosmos.

Those of you who don't know anything about me,

I'll begin by telling you.

A G-O-D, that's what I gotta be.

I can't be a mortal living immortality.

Don't drop yo Guard.

Let the Dead Rize.

The Rebirth will take place right before your eyes.

I used to always think about suicide.

Now I'm thinking of ways to help me stay alive.

That's why I give my thanks and praises

To the MOST HIGH.

Because the MOST HIGH will decide when I die.

I try to eat right; try to live right;

And consistently pray for DIVINE INSIGHT.

The soul of the Trinity

Lives within you, lives within me.

I look at death like the sick looks at health.

I feel the feeling when the feeling's being felt.

I step wit pride; speak wit determination.

Wit JAH as my guide, I have the motivation

To move mountains and build a new nation.

ANCESTORS' anticipation gives me inspiration

To really just "BE"

And develop the powers GOD has given me.

I acknowledge GOD shares ITS powers wit I.

I pray for TRUE GUIDANCE 'til the day I die.

Measurements of motion verify time.

In our measurements of motion,

We need a Peace of Mind.

A Peace of Mind, A Peace of Mind

Is all we have in a lifetime.

A Peace of Mind is hard to get

But it's much harder to keep it.

It may be easier to be conceited.

Our spirits have a cosmological blueprint

Based on knowledge, wisdom, and common sense.

Our Knowledge tells us four quarters is a dollar.

Our Wizdom tells us how to spend a dollar.

Common sense balances the two.

Without common sense, we would all be through.

Simplicity is the simplest form of order.

So many are out of order they praise martyrs.

When you choose the way you live,

You decide how you die.

Living in vain is a shame, no lie.

I get high through my meditation and prayers.

Truth or Dare, the M.P.E.R.O.R. really cares.

A Peace of Mind. . . many may seek this.

Some people may take my kindness for weakness.

My kindness is where my strength comes from.

I rhyme this wit intent of the outcome

To reach people who are deaf,

Dumb and blind.

You will hear, speak, see

When you have Peace of Mind.

A Peace of Mind, A Peace of Mind
Is all we have in a lifetime.

I do what I can when I can when I have it.
This universe is built
Off the science of mathematics.
Mathematics is the language of the universe.
I have to be a zero before I am the first.
When I multiply, add, and divide
The things I minus,
I'm laying the foundation
Which will elevate science.
We can't stop the development of technology.
We need spiritual dimensions in the psychology
To learn how to maintain
And keep the scales balanced.
Develop our talents;
Deal wit challenge
By the gallons.
Opposition will test you, but help you try.
If it wasn't for the wind, a bird wouldn't fly.

If it wasn't for success,

There would be no struggle.

The resistance of weights help manifest yo muscle.

Building blocks of each cell will compel

To bring us together if all else fails.

From plants to planets, Francis Welsing has landed.

The enterprise of the Mothership

Has been granted.

Now, I chanted

Go for self and demand it.

Command it not to be abandoned.

God makes decisions when man plans it.

We're spiritual beings

Passing through a human transit.

And it may seem that we are stranded

On this asphalt desert we have been branded

To be a gangsta, outlaw, or bandit.

I'm Frank like Sinatra because I'm candid.

The teachings of OUR ANCESTORS

Have been Xpanded.

This time around, these devils cannot band it.

Life is what you make it, so I make this life mine.

THE CREATOR has helped me to have
A Peace of Mind.

For one to search for one's soul
In the world is an illusion.
There is no peace on the outside of you.
The only peace you have is on the inside.
Don't let no one take that peace.
A Peace of Mind — that's all I got.

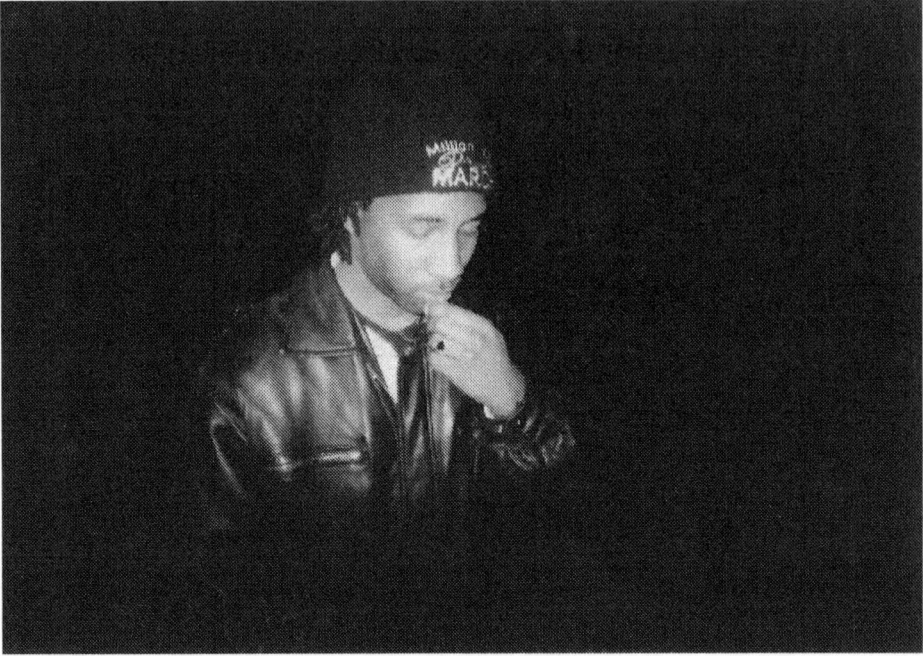

Track 4

Track 4 is about one of many near death xperiences I've had. I say one of many not to be arrogant, but to be appreciative. See, in my eyes, anytime we are conscious of something happening and then know that we could have died from what happened, that is a near death xperience. Afterward, you make a transition from being consciously aware into being aware of your conscience.

Every time we close our eyes to sleep and then wake up, we have had a near death xperience. To eat our food unaware of the digestive system process is a near death xperience. I and i can go on and on.

"When a king sleeps, he forgets about his palace. When a prisoner sleeps, he forgets about the prison," said Hazrat Khan.

Some people have asked me why this lesson is entitled *Track 4*. I could get into some astrological, metaphysical, geocentric science about the letters of the word "track" and the number "4," but honestly, at the time I recorded, I didn't have a name for it and it was the forth lesson I recorded. So it was titled *Track 4*. Now, the type of font that was used makes the "4" look like the letter "U." Once again, I could go into "Yo, the font makes the number four look like the letter U. So, the forces beyond were conveying the lesson as 'Track U' cuz OUR ANCESTORS keep us on track." Yo, it ain't that deep! Just one of dem things.

GUIDANCE

Track 4

Yo, Yo! Just wanted to thank everybody who got the CD. Everyone who's been supporting me for the last years. I and i truly appreciate your support.

On January 29, 2000, I got behind the wheel of my car with a very foul spirit. It was one of those days when it was snowing. There was ice on the roads. Well, I was on the highway and I was in the fast lane, tripping. Like I said, I had a very foul spirit cuz I had some things on my mental, you know. Well, I hit a piece of ice and my car hit the median and spun around, hit the median again, and just died – just stayed there.

I was thinking to myself that I needed to get to the ditch. There weren't any cars coming . . . yet. As I had that thought, it was like the GREAT FORCE started coasting my car over to the ditch.

Well, as it was coasting, I was trying to get out of the car to look behind me. It's like it was happening and it wasn't happening. That was when I knew I was between the two worlds.

As I got into the middle of the lane, there was an 18-wheeler coming behind me. As it rapidly approached me, I gave the yell of death "AHHHHHHHHHHHH!!!" The GREAT FORCE stopped my car . . . the 18-wheeler passed and I was guided to the ditch.

One of my brothuz came to pick me up (Min Truth – Tizir Smith). They say a lesson not learned will be repeated. For me, the lesson was: she had gone on living her life and you need to keep living yours.

Once, there was a man walking in the jungle. He saw a tiger. The tiger started chasing him. The man took off running down a cliff until he saw a vine and started climbing down the vine. When he looked down the vine, he saw two lions waiting for him. So, he started climbing back up. When he looked up, he saw that there was a rat nibbling on the vine. He looked across from where he was and saw a strawberry. He reached for the strawberry and took a bite out if it. It was the sweetest strawberry he had ever tasted in his life!

The lesson: when the man realized he was in a situation he could not control, he took time to enjoy the simplest, sweetest part of life. Don't Let No One Take Away Your Strawberry!

TRUE GUIDANCE

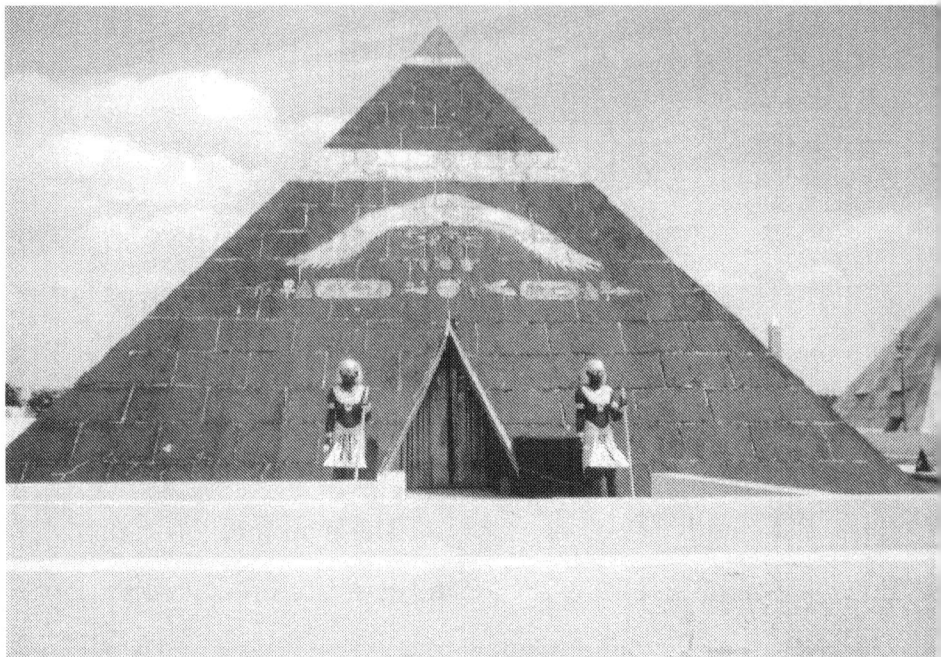

Aum Vam Dhum

Aum Vam Dhum is the first meditation I learned studying with the Ausar Auset Society. Ausar is the Afrikan name for Osiris and Auset is the Afrikan name for Isis, each representing the masculine and feminine powers, respectively. Auset is known to be the mother of Earth/living. She is the nurturer, provider, protector, and, of course, the healer. Every man needs a woman who is a healer.

The words "Aum Vam Dhum" do not have a meaning, but the vibrations of these words speak volumes of the soundless sound. The universal sound is ohm or aum, but we know it best as um.

I have xperienced so many of my most meaningful expressions from this particular meditation. Jasmine is one of the fragrances used to enhance the trance. To this day, the scent of Jasmine always puts me into a trance. It reminds me of the inner peace I've become acquainted with as well as reminds me of how I must protect that peace.

The third verse of this lesson is what I said to a Queen when I and i proposed to her. When I tell people this, they often ask me what she said. So, for those of you who want to know her answer, she said no. When I asked her why, she said she didn't love me anymore.

We had been apart for a year, but she was still in my veins. We communicated during the break-up. Just as there is a process of getting to know a person, there is a process of letting the person go.

I have this ting (thing) about being older and looking back at my life. If I didn't propose to her, I would have regretted never knowing how she would respond, you know. It was mad peace. My Queen Mother helped me pick out the ring, but I took it back by myself (smile). When I told my King Father, his only words were, "She did you a favor."

Respect!

Aum Vam Dhum

Our deepest fear is not that we're inadequate. Our deepest fear is that we are powerful beyond measure. It is our light, not our darkness that frightens us. We ask ourselves "Who am I to be brilliant, gorgeous, talented and fabulous?" Actually, who are you not to be?

- Nelson Mandela

Aum Vam Dhum

Queen of all Queens; Goddess born Goddess.

Appearance is modest; foundation is honest.

Relationship platonic, vibing off erotic.

You and yours have wisdom; I and i have knowledge.

We come together to balance the two.

Without you there's no me;

Without me there's no you.

Dear sistah, women aren't women no more.

Instead of being a highness,

They want to be a whore.

Black women, I give them their respect.

But when they don't respect they self,

They need to check they self.

I can't believe they let they self neglect they self.

They wreck they self

Cause they never met they self.

If they only knew the Auset and unveiled Isis

Then they might just become righteous.

Eternal love, everlasting athletic,

Agile with her child speaking Kemetic.

Aum Vam Dhum, Aum Vam Dhum

Twa ankh nut sa en ankh auset tum

Dear sistah, a divine lesson.

Thank you Auset, essence of life your love blessing.

Queen, you showed me that I'm destined

To fulfill the prophesy

The ancients were addressing.

You showed me how to turn a house into a home.

And when I felt lonely, your reminded me

I'm not alone.

Aum Vam Dhum, Auh Vam Dhum

Twa ankh nut sa en ankh auset tum

Aum Vam Dhum, Auh Vam Dhum

I am the King Sun - You are the Queen Moon.

Black woman, so much has happened between us.

Unfortunately, distrust is stronger than trust.

In ancient times, our souls were parallel,

But now, we're under this Willie Lynch spell.

Light vs. Dark; Old vs. Young

Short vs. Tall; Knowledge vs. Wisdom.

Conquer by dividing our divine attributes.

Every time we meet, we have these bad attitudes.

The M.P.E.R.O.R. has to take a stand.

You have fake hair, fake eyes, fake nails

Yet you want a real man.

Sistahs are hurting; brothas are hurting,

Our children are hurting. We haven't been working

Up to our fullest potential towards elevation.

Heed the ancients' credentials of our creation.

A nation within a nation building

With strength, humbleness, and patience healing

The mind, body, soul with alchemy.

In our mental balcony there's spiritual faculty

That governs our life force on our life course.

Even in life, sports don't pay to take life shorts.

What goes around comes around.

You reap what you sow.

Throughout the earth, throughout the cosmos,

We must grow

In love and make our hearts lighter than a feather.

Marry to Maat Tua Neter

Aum Vam Dhum, Aum Vam Dhum

Twa ankh nut sa en ankh auset tum

Aum Vam Dhum, Aum Vam Dhum

I am the King Sun - You are the Queen Moon.

Black woman, Goddess of All and All.

I remember the writings on the wall

To sketch you out to be the universe.

Black woman represents heaven on earth.

When you hear me chant

Aum Vam Dhum

It's just a reminder that sun reflects

With the moon.

On the other side of the mountains of the moon,

In the valley of beginnings is where I consume.

You are the justice I must protect

With my life, tears, blood,

but most of all, my sweat.

Mental loving is needed; spiritual loving is a must.

Physical hugging is greeted with trust.

You got my back and I got yours

Through the thunder and lightening the rain pours.

The love in my heart has been carved with a knife.

Queen, I know you my wife,

However, I walk patiently on my mission.

Remembering man makes plans,

But God makes decisions.

If it's gon be, it's gon be.

Keep in mind, Queen, Freedom Ain't Free.

The Great Sacrifice will come forth

And bring together west, east, south, and north.

Hotepu Neteru

The M.P.E.R.O.R. needs a Goddess Guru.

Aum Vam Dhum, Aum Vam Dhum

Twa ankh nut sa en ankh auset tum

Aum Vam Dhum, Aum Vam Dhum

I am the King Sun - You are the Queen Moon.

- Talk (Aum Vam Dhum) -

Queen Wisdom Asiatic, all we have is one another. Don't let no one tear us apart. Without you, I am nothing. With you, I can conquer the world.

Everything is everything.

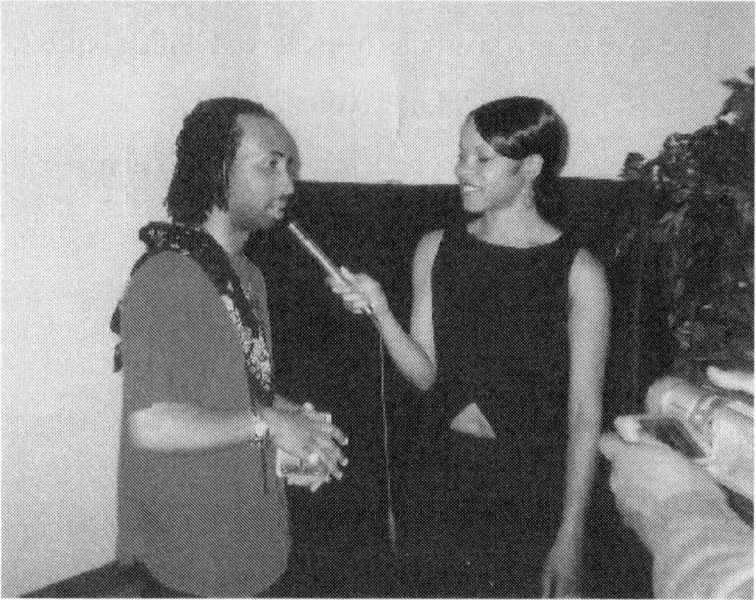

Parting

You and I assumed forever

When we became companions.

But now, unhappy, you are leaving.

The sky turns to bitter candescence

Unslaked by resignation.

There are times when we have been lucky enough to have companions on our spiritual path, but the time of parting often comes without welcome. When our friends decide to leave, we are often left with doubt, confusion, and sometimes guilt.

Anyone may leave the path. They won't suffer damnation; they will only walk a different path.

The rule for those who follow Tao is this: Walk the path together as long as you can, and when you must part, never hold your companion back.

Should one seek to have no feelings at all regarding friends? After all, the sages constantly warn us against attachment. Yet emotion is part of what makes us human. We may understand philosophically why a companion must leave, but we need not deny our feelings as we walk on alone.* When you drink water, remember the source.

*This passage taken from 365 TAO.

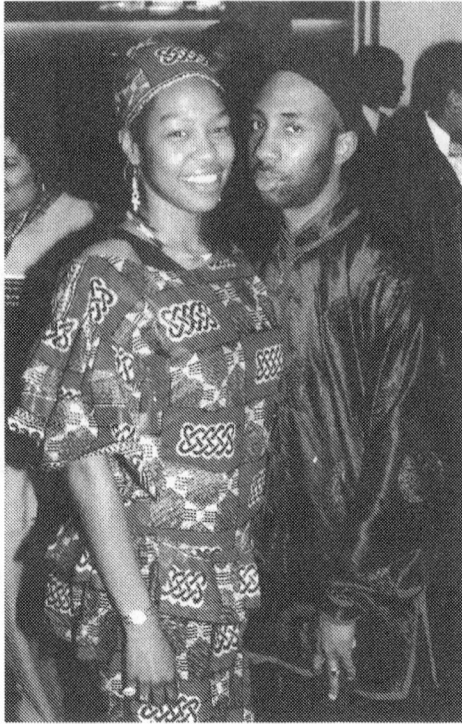

Jah's Divine Light

This lesson is about my X-wisdom. How we met, how we lived and shared our xperiences with each other. How we parted.

I remember meditating on the lesson and seeing the performance. I always saw her (my X-wisdom) in the audience.

Well, the night I decided to go to an open mic to manifest this lesson, she walked in with another cat (man). Yo, my heart dropped. I was going to leave right then, but I couldn't. "This walk" was greater than I could imagine.

With the spiritual powers I was developing, I and i manifested like never before. It was definitely a classic M.P.E.R.O.R. performance. Seeing her with this other cat, friend or not, was reality smacking me in the face. That was definitely one of the best tings (things) that happened to me. But yo, it hurt like a muddaphukka.

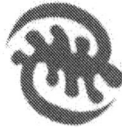

Once, there was a warrior who was fighting for THE CREATOR/GOD. He and his enemy were banging to the death. The warrior had gotten the best of his enemy and was about to finish him off. So, he pulled out his sword to cut of his enemy's head. As he raised his sword, his enemy spat in the warriors face. This was all the warrior's enemy had in him.

The warrior wiped the spit off his face, put his sword back in the holster, and walked away. He walked away because once he got spat on, it became personal. He was no longer fighting for THE CREATOR, but for himself.

It's crazy hard at times not to take things personally. I took it personally when my X-wisdom came to the club with another cat. My performance was greater than hers and his.

The lesson is greater than I could ever imagine. JAH's DIVINE LIGHT is the most requested song/lesson off *Tribute To The Black Woman.*

Blessed Be

Jah's Divine Light

We started out meeting at the Xpo.

I came to see you perform at yo next show.

You were doing your ting-ting, dancing and singing.

I dug what you were bringing and swinging.

My secret status and mysterious aura

Had you captivated like the Holy Torah.

Queen, I truly adore you – wanted more of you.

You know the routine

When I would open the door for you.

Any time we entered a building, I entered first.

The Black Man must protect

The Black Mother Earth.

It's the least I can do, Queen,

For having me at birth.

Black Woman, you're my heaven.

I know what you're worth –

More than diamonds, gold or any minerals.

Divide the universe by two and

We're the individuals.

At times we chill.

Other times we ill.

But every time we build,

I felt that spiritual appeal.

I felt this was gonna be alright;

You felt this was gonna be alrigh;t

We felt this was gonna be alright;

We're replicas of JAH'S DIVINE LIGHT.

I felt this was gonna be alright;

You felt this was gonna be alright;

We felt this was gonna be alrigh;t

We're replicas of JAH'S DIVINE LIGHT.

A couple of months down the line,

Things were going fine.

A couple of months after that,

They started to decline.

We're arguing just a little too much.

Is it real lust, fake love, or God's true touch?

We both had baggage from our past relationships,

Then we brought it into this relationship.

You pulled my patience slip,

Always questioning my loyalty.

The lie I told you

Protected the truth of my royalty.

We break up to make up,

Now how long will this last?

We both had a problem

Getting the past to be the past.

You prayed for a God man, I manifest.

I prayed for a Queen. You became my Goddess.

We both met our match with each other.

I'm more than a man and your friend, sistah,

I'm your brotha.

Justice is Divine when the scales are balanced.

My silence was your main challenge.

I felt this was gonna be alright;

You felt this was gonna be alright;

We felt this was gonna be alright;

We're replicas of JAH'S DIVINE LIGHT.

Yo, things are gonna be alright;

In a minute, it's all gon be alright;

JAH knows it's all gon be alright;

Cuz we're replicas of JAH's DIVINE LIGHT.

Yo, things are gonna be alright;

In a minute, it's all gon be alright;

JAH knows it's all gon be alright;

Cuz we're replicas of JAH's DIVINE LIGHT.

Our love was an xzample for our people.

I was your other half and you were my equal.

The arguments and the drama was so petty.

I snapped at you steady, but through silence

You could have met me.

We both feel we need space right.

Went to the oracles and now it's verified.

It's hard to let go and let GOD purify.

If it's meant to be, it'll be . . . .the other side.

I felt like I lost a sacred treasure.

A couple of weeks after we parted,

Your dad became an ANCESTOR.

I wanted to be there; you didn't want me near.

A panther in rage trapped in a cage.

You went from saying you wanted space
To you needed your freedom.
From the glossary to the index is how I read 'em.
Freedom Ain't Free. Freedom Ain't Free.
Sometimes you have to lose your eye sight
Just to see.
Rain beats down on a leopard,
But it doesn't wash away the spots.
The love we have for each other won't stop.
I'll keep you in my prayers.
See you when you get there
And be your silent protector while you're here.

I felt this was gonna be alright;
You felt this was gonna be alright;
We felt this was gonna be alright;
We're replicas of JAH'S DIVINE LIGHT.

- Talk -

The only way a diamond becomes a diamond is by the
pressure of the coal. The only way you polish a diamond is by

using friction. The pressure you may be dealing with in this society and the friction you may be dealing with from different people means THE CREATOR is only polishing you to shine as bright as a diamond.

That's Word!

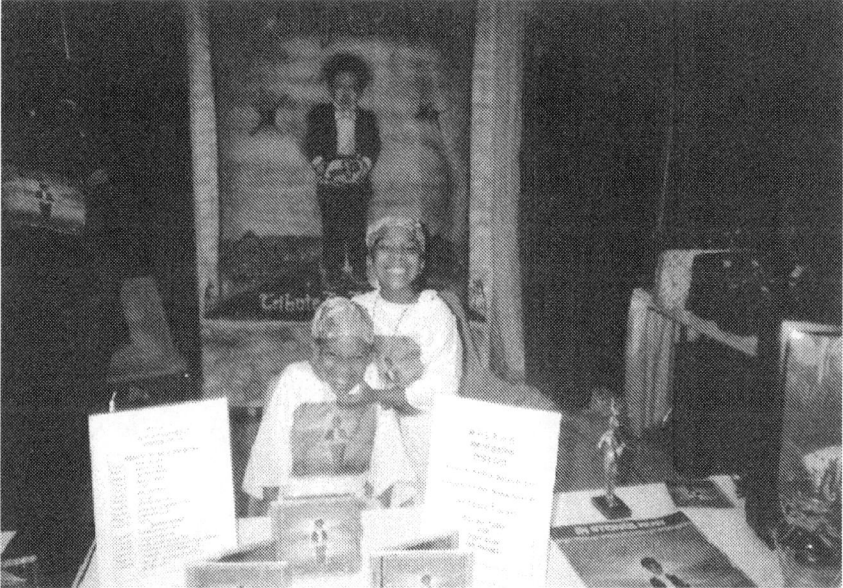

Justice is Divine (Intro)

We are an Afrikan people

Robbed of our homeland.

Robbed of our name.

Robbed of our brotherhood, our sisterhood,

Our motherhood, our fatherhood,

Our nationhood, our religion.

We shall rise

Never to fall again.

Up You Mighty People!

We can accomplish what we will.

No Justice – No Peace.

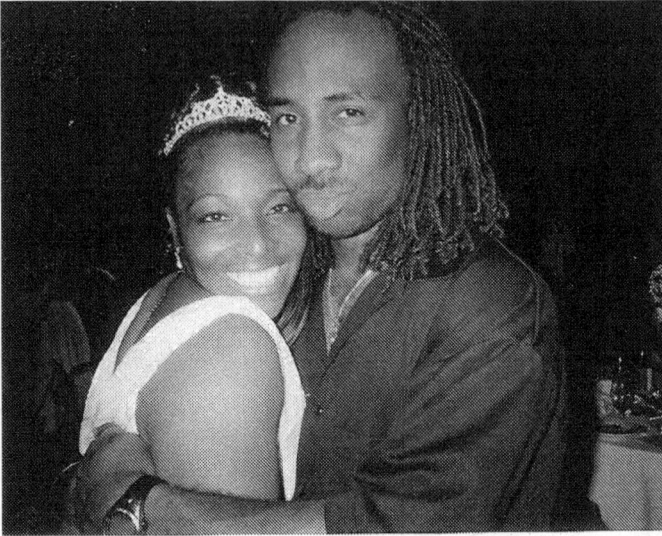

Justice Is Divine

In Ancient Africa, a woman named Maat represents Justice. She has a blindfold over her eyes, holding a scale. On one side of the scale is your heart. On the other side is a feather. The question is, "Is your heart heavier or lighter than a feather? If it is heavier, what must you do to make it lighter?"

In this great country of Amerikkka, the goal is to resemble Ancient Afrika, only Amerikkka lacks the morals. Let knowledge be born. They have a woman representing justice (which was stolen from Ancient Afrika), yet constantly degrade, exploit, and treat women like old furniture. Even the White woman has to fight her White man for imaginary equality. For the sake of the Earth dwellers' sanity, note: I and i are speaking in general.

Sex and violence sells. There was a time when sex was sacred and violence was for liberation. In some places, this may still be. For the most part, sex is not respected and violence is at will.

"You have great warriors who are steadfast, prayerful, and meditative for the day of. There is no honor for the day of . . . nowadays. There are many teachers, but the fearlessness disciples are very few" (I AM THAT).

Justice Is Divine is simply about "justice" being represented by a woman.

"There's nothing new under the sun." – King Solomon.

In ancient Africa, the Black woman (Maat) was looked upon and respected as justice. Now, the Black woman must see herself, love and respect herself as justice. As Black men, we must see the Black woman and love and respect her as justice.

Have you ever heard the words "No Justice – No Peace?" Let us examine these words.

Brothaz, have you ever been with a woman and everything was right and xzact? The way she talked to you, the way she healed you, the way she cooked, cleaned, conversed with you? It's just something about a woman's touch. Granted, we all have had some messed up xperiences, but just try to remember the good times for this particular exercise.

Brothaz, what was good was that she brought justice to our turmoil. When we thought there was no peace in war, she was our peace. Give thanks for the lesson and remember, "No Justice – No Peace."

Justice is Divine

What happens in the dark is revealed to the light.

I whisper, "Move closer. I don't bite."

A blazing chill runs down my spine.

And you are on my mind?

As we start to touch lips, our thoughts combine.

Not a pity in my soul. My heart's filled with joy.

I'm too much of a man to be treated like a boy,

So don't tease me in order to please me.

Perfection can't be rushed,

So let's take it slow and easy.

I not only understand,

I overstand what you tell me.

That's why I leave

That bump and grind stuff to R. Kelly.

I'm here even after the physical urges are gone.

When I'm afraid, my fear is my courage.

As we grow together, we're no longer lost sheep.

Like the trees on the planet earth,

Our roots run deep.

We must know ourselves to manifest the fruits.

If we don't know ourselves,

We're like a tree without its roots —

Unable to grow, unable to live,

Unable to destroy the negative

And build the positive.

All we have is one another.

I'm more than a man and a friend,

Sistah, I'm your brotha.

What we have is genuine.

When the scales are balanced,

Our Justice is Divine.

I walk through the swamp

To reach the valley of the streams.

I walk along the Nile

And think about what I've seen.

Let knowledge be born like water runs in a creek.

Dreams only come to people who are asleep.

I don't dream upon making a decision.

The sleeper has awakened with a vision.

I have 180 degrees of knowledge for the better.

The 360 won't be completed until we're together.

The trust and love is gone,

So we must re-establish it.

On one solid foundation,

We build our establishment.

Teach what we know to those who don't know.

I thank the MOST HIGH for my soul

And thank the Nile for my flow.

Our current capacity travels

Throughout the universe

As we represent the true and living

On this planet earth.

I am because we are.

Because we are,

Therefore I am.

A courageous, brave and wise man.

Even with a clock, people still can't tell time.

No Justice, No Peace.

With peace our Justice is Divine.

People who pray together stay together.

Join me in prayer and make our hearts lighter

Than a feather.

We give thanks and praises to THE MOST HIGH.

The same things that make us smile

Will make us cry.

We can move mountains with your assistance.

Live through our souls

And bring forth a character of your xzistence.

Guide and protect us to stay on a righteous path.

Make us aware of any ignorance we may have.

So our indwelling intelligence will manifest

And we can be wise and civilize on our quest

For freedom, justice, and equality.

Our cosmology is a divine policy

Of truth and righteousness

In the ways of the scale.

We're standing at the crossroads

'Cuz we've been through Hell.

We must get to the other side.

Allow our lessons in life to serve as our guide

To destroying the negative

And building the positive.

We're making a life out of living as we live.

So many are lost. When they seek, they shall find.

When we come together, our Justice is Divine.

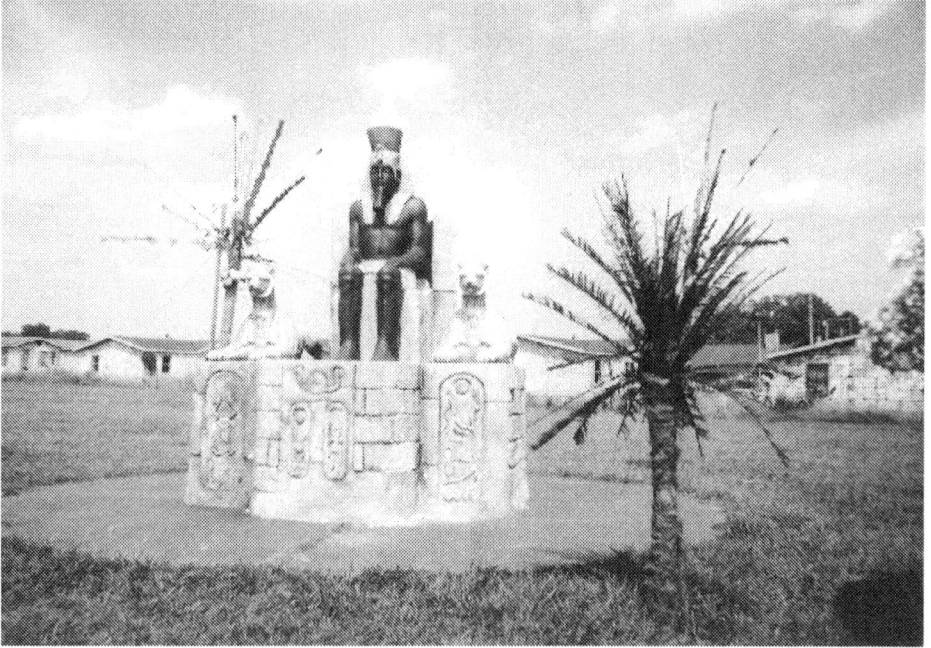

Justice is Divine (outro)

If you study the relationship between the slave master and the slave, you discover a similar relationship between the Black man and the Black woman. We degrade our women. We exploit our women. It has gotten so bad that sistahs have started turning to other sistahs for comfort.

See, brothaz, when you give a woman a house, she'll make it into a home. When you give a woman food, she'll make it into a meal. When you give a woman your seed, she'll manifest your child. Let knowledge be born!

The M.P.E.R.O.R. Royal L is a spiritual uplifter.

Man is a life giver.

The woman is a life bearer, it is clear.

The M.P.E.R.O.R. promotes meditation and prayer.

Forget the egos. It takes a woman and a man

To bring forth future and walk across this land.

So brothuz, relieve the egos and confess.

Sistahs, put your pride aside to progress.

Many relationships are like serving a life sentence.

Ask yourself if your spouse

Is a help or a hindrance.

If they're a hindrance, you're living on death row.

When I was on death row, I always felt low.

I was holding on to someone who wasn't there.

It was like holding on to the air.

Like a mortal, I was screaming, "Life isn't fair!"

Little did I know, I was being prepared.

See, while she was making me a man under the sun,

God was molding me into the man I've become.

Now, I'm God-Body focus to the max.

A Peace of Mind helps my soul to relax.

I admit, I have a long way to go

But my rhythmic rapping coincides

With the Nile's Flow.

And yo, before I G-O,

The best way to keep someone you love

Is to simply let 'em go.

Fly like an eagle.

No matter what, I'll die with my people.

If they don't return,

They weren't yours from the start.

That's coming straight from the heart

Of the M.P.E.R.O.R.

Da Da Da Da Daaaaaaaaaaaaaaaaa . . .

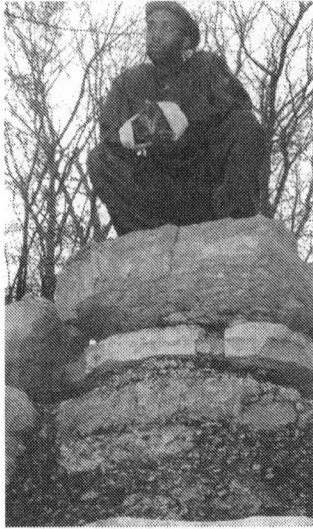

T.R.M.

"The Righteous Man" is probably one of the most creative lessons I've done. It's a style I always wanted to do. I and i refer to this style as doo-wop hip-hop. My brother Steve "God Man" Ward sang four part harmonies a cappella as I rapped over the harmonies.

The lesson is geared toward the so-called "Enlightened Ones." These are the ones who are not only consciously aware, but who are also aware of their conscious. These are the people who have chosen the path of the pure versus the path of the unsure.

"You have realized that you are one of the Original Sons or Daughters of God. This must not be taken lightly. This realization is one of the keys to our people's liberation."

- The Late, Great Professor X of X-Clan

T.R.M.

When I came into this world, I had nothing to give.

I cried when I came alive and I'm crying as I live.

Sometimes, it's hard to live righteous.

I need proper guidance.

I already know I'm gonna die in this.

We were all born to die.

When I walk, I walk with my head towards the sky.

Timely situations purify my third eye.

The same things that make me smile

Will make me cry.

As I make a life out of living

A simple and complete lifestyle,

I walk the banks and learn the lessons

In the waters of the Nile.

I may often get stressed and be depressed.

These are the times when I bring forth my best.

I've overcome many obstacles in my path.

When I overcome the obstacles,

I sit back and laugh.

Then I trip on how something had me up for grabs.

I dig deep within myself to find the genetic maps

That guide me in the right direction.

My suggestion is to ask more questions.

When you feel you can't talk to anyone else,

You'll always find the answer in your true self.

So I live to love – love to live like a star,

Shining bright the guiding light

Through the night Anuk Ausar.

Many are just a carbon copy,

But I'm the true and living

Manifestation of God-Body.

You can't keep a Black man down

You can't keep a Black man down

You can't keep a Black man down

You can't keep a Black man down

You can't keep a Black woman down

You can't keep a Black woman down

You can't keep a Black woman down

You can't keep a Black woman down

It's a miraculous miracle

Manifested in the physical.

The mental is spiritual; the left side is analytical.

The right side is guidance

Toward the opening of the way.

It takes seconds, minutes, hours,

Just to make up a day.

When I pray, there's no limit upon my xzistence.

My motivation has made

My determination consistent.

I am persistent. Ice Cube has told you,

I'm not the one.

I xpect what occurs cuz I anticipate the outcome.

I'm the M.P.E.R.O.R.,

The tree of life that bears fruit.

In order to know truth, you must live in truth.

Through prayer and meditation

I live in true guidance.

My King Father is fine;

My Queen Mother is the finest.

My Earthly parents are responsible for my birth.

God made it possible for me to live on Earth.

Goddess gave my mother nourishment in the event.

My earthly father can't believe

He had God-Body in his semen.

Now, I'm a living form of the light; I'm the brightest.

Despite this ignorance, I try to live righteous.

So, I'm building every second, minute, hour,

Gaining more spiritual power.

I had to die to the things of the world.

Now I've risen from the dead.

My body no longer controls my head.

I'm the master of my world. I'm even with the odd.

A temptation from the devil is a test by God.

So check it, I'm guided and protected.

I've been selected

To be the cause behind the cause

Of what's being affected.

I'm the blessed to make the unblessed confess it.

A wise man compromises, a fool would test it.

A man's life was already written, I check it.

There's no such thing

As coincidence and accidents.

I wrecked it.

Pain is a part of life.

I feel and I've felt it.

Living in misery is a choice,

But don't accept it.

My mind is a mirror

Where your true self is reflected.

Be true to yourself, real with yourself

And don't neglect it.

I'm connected with the DIVINE, I'm respected.

Now, I can't rest in peace

Cuz I've been resurrected.

You can't keep a Black man down

You can't keep a Black man down

You can't keep a Black man down

You can't keep a Black man down

You can't keep a Black woman down

You can't keep a Black woman down

You can't keep a Black woman down

You can't keep a Black woman down

You can't keep the Black people down
You can't keep the Black people down
You can't keep the Black people down
You can't keep the Black people down

You can't keep the Black Folk down
You can't keep the Black Folk down
You can't keep the Black Folk down
You can't keep the Black Folk down

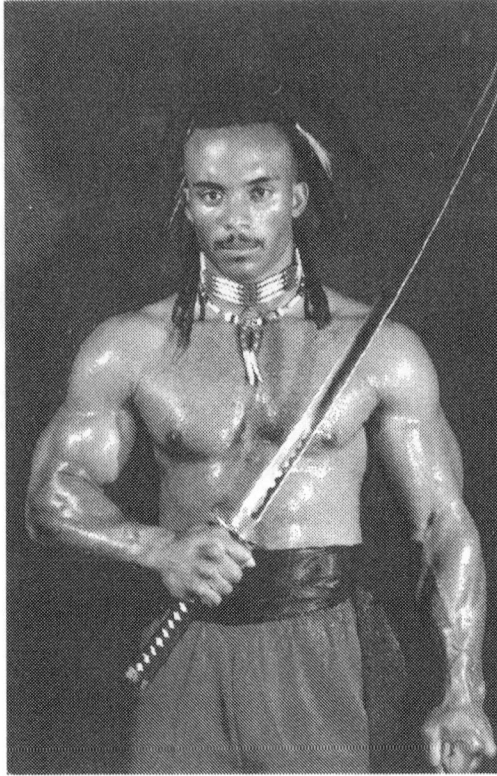

Last Testimony of G.O.D.

Many moons ago, I began a quest for knowledge, wisdom and overstanding. Everyone in this life tends to come to the point on the road where we ask ourselves the question, "Who am I?"

I remember, once upon a time, asking, "Why me? Why me?" It seemed like things of uncertainty always happened to me. One day, in frustration and anger, I asked, "Why me?" My inner voice answered, "Why not you?"

I then began learning that whenever you pray for strength, humility, patience, knowledge, wisdom, and overstanding, you are asking for the circumstances that enable you to become consciously aware of such things. Once you begin to put those things in practice, you become aware of your conscience.

The Bible says, "Many are called, but few are chosen." These words often used to puzzle me. We're all taught that GOD doesn't have any favoritism, but these words seem to prove that teaching wrong. As a student of Shekem Ur Shekem Ra Un Nefer Amen, I find the words "Many are called but few are chosen" simply to mean: "Many will call upon GOD, but few will choose to live in TRUTH" (Metu Neter, Vol. 2).

When the question is asked to our Grand Master Teacher (PBUH) Hazrat Inyat Khan, "How can you tell when a person knows God?" he answers, "A person who knows GOD is not one who is always talking about GOD, but one whose silence says it."

I have been blessed to study with some of the greatest master and grand master teachers not known to the masses. I have been even more blessed in learning how to apply the sacred teachings of OUR ANCESTORS to everyday challenges in life. I can see why THE MOST HIGH came to the planet before his Son and personally destroyed Sodom and Gomorrah (Gen. 19-25). I overstand why THE MOST HIGH struck people down with lightening.

I was told once before that if you really want to not just "understand" the Bible, but have an "overstanding" of the Bible, whenever you see Jesus's name in the Bible, put your name in its place.

The Bible speaks of God never destroying the world again. God doesn't have to destroy the world again because the people of the world will destroy themselves. Look how easy we justify what we know is wrong.

The norm for the masses is living to eat instead of eating to live. These words – living to eat – speak volumes. Living to eat not only means food, but it also means keeping up with the Joneses, the paper chase, the fast pace of living, etc.

Our beloved brother Bob Marley (PBUH) once said, "You can't stop the development of technology." In ancient times, the focus was teaching people to become better people. In these times, the focus is teaching people to make better things.

Let knowledge be born! When the focus is on teaching people to become better people, it is only natural for better things to come about.

The *Last Testimony of GOD* is about my spiritual development in not only becoming a man of God, but being God Man.

Last Testimony of G.O.D.

I am the one who transforms into two.

I am two who transforms into four.

I am four who transforms into eight.

After this, I am one.

If there is no test, then there is no testimony.

Sometimes I feel that I am the only

One who goes through the things I grow through.

Father-Mother GOD said

Those things will mold you.

I hold you with the heart I owe you.

I told you your part will scold you.

Move with the earth; xperience days and nights.

Move with the sun; you will only know light.

Out of darkness comes light.

No matter how dark it gets in your life

You can make it bright.

Greater within me than in the world.

Greater within me will end the world.

Greater within me may offend the world.

With the message Greater within me

Sends the world.

There are many thorns but few flowers.

Study and develop spiritual powers.

Rhythmic Rain dances rain showers.

The ones you thought were courageous

Were cowards.

Heart and will are driven by desire.

Don't turn your cheek

Against the double-minded liars.

I and i bring brimstone and fire.

It gets deeper and deeper; higher and higher.

While some are singing in the choir,

People like myself make devils retire.

Storm the gate; tear down the empire.

Born to take what we had prior . . . FREEDOM.

To whom much is given, much is required.

I applied for the job, but I was already hired.

M.P.E.R.O.R. Royal Lord Black Rap Messiah.

Spiritual uplifter; TRUE GUIDANCE supplier.

Brainwash individuals, I am the dryer.

They want me to sell my soul,

But find another buyer.

People have problems with things I transpire.

Still the man among men they admire.

In a few days, this life will xpire.

Flesh is the Siren – Spirit is the Sire.

When the Word became flesh,

I was told this life could cause stress.

It's a mess. Sometimes I get depressed.

When I give my best, G-Force does the rest.

It's a lonely road on the path of the pure.

Only God knows what I endure.

When my flesh doubts, my spirit stays sure.

The masses are asses. They've been allured!

Lost in fantasy and confusion.

To search for your soul in the world is an illusion.

I and i come with spiritual intrusion.

He-is-a-dog.com is part of my persecution.

Sometimes I wonder,

Why do they want to take me under?

People want rain without thunder.

A poor and a rich man both feel hunger.

Who will out fox the fox?

Put the cornerstone where they build blocks.

Knowledge of self; the master key to the locks.

When the game is over,

Kings and pawns go in the same box.

This is just a mere milestone.

Give me an inch and we can take it a mile long.

Don't worry about what this child's on.

To mama, I'm a baby.

To this world, I'm a child grown.

Don't nobody love me like mama.

My father's tough love helps me

Deal with the drama.

I'm a survivor through trauma.

M.P.E.R.O.R. the Dalai Lama.

In Arabic, I'm the Great Mahdi.

I am that, I am that be God-Lee.

In Rastafari, you know JAH-BE.

Most High in Hebrew is who YAH-BE.

Conquering Lion and tribe of Judah.

Christ the Savior me lives the life of Buddah.

Praise be to GOD or HalleluYAH.

Or HalleluJAH, Peace to ALLAH.

My spirit transcends my Ka to the Ba.

My Kundalini signifies Amon-Ra.

What you have seen I already saw.

Reverse my orgasm, create like PTAH.

King of Kings; Lord of Lords.

My disciple stays strapped with guns,

Bombs, knives and swords.

I got guards, you got guards.

Any man can be touched in and out of the yards.

Storm of life must be weathered

By making your heart lighter than a feather.

One man's trash is another's treasure.

Many lives have been ruined

For a moment of pleasure.

When you wake up and the sun don't shine,

You become conscious that you're blind.

Mother Nature and Father Time

Made it clear that my lethal weapon is my mind.

The brain is the perfect storehouse for wealth.

The path of the pure is the path to health.

Like a thief in the night, learn to move in stealth.

This is the last testimony of the Guerilla of Death.

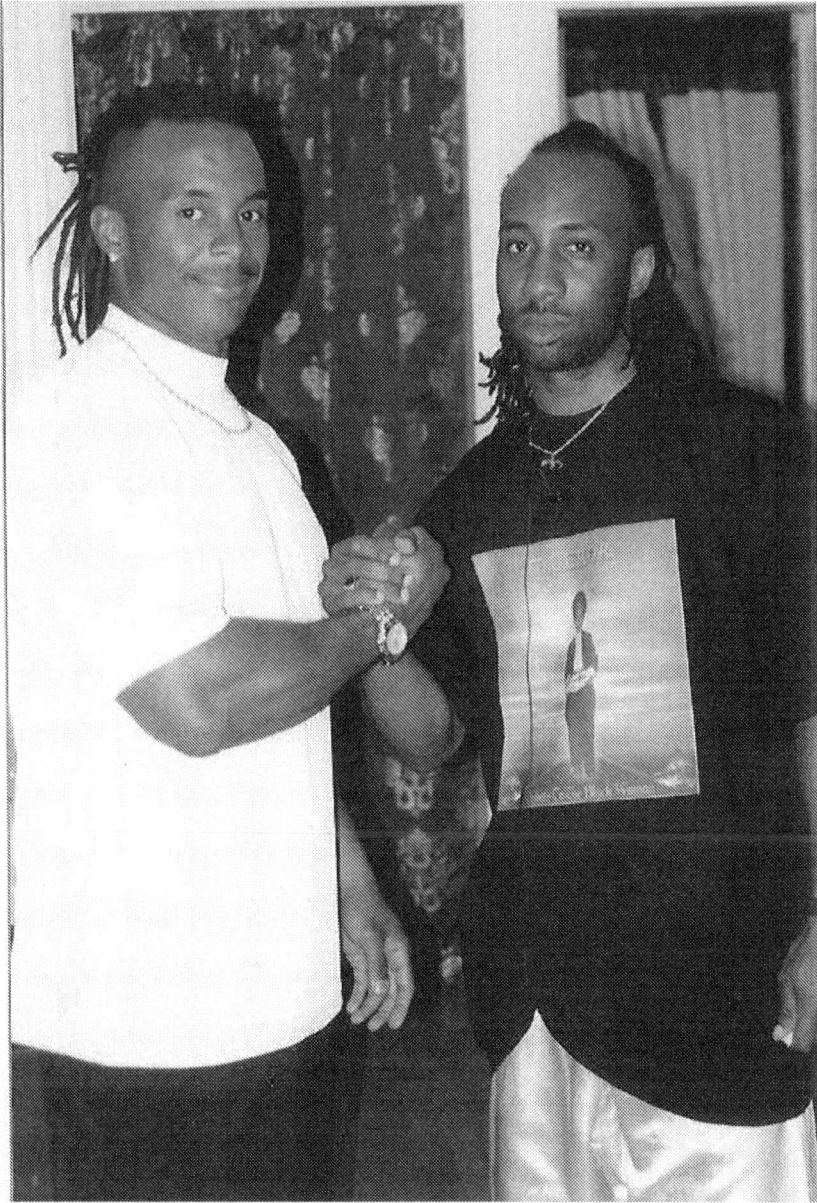

Assisting women spiritually as well as mentally and emotionally, respectively, are: World Champion Cage Fighter Jermaine "Bam Bam" Andre and M.P.E.R.O.R.

References

Afua, Q. (1991). *Heal Thyself.* Brooklyn, NY: A&B Publisher Group.

Amen, R. (1990). *Metu Neter, Vol. 1.* New York, NY: Khamit Corporation.

Amen, R. (1990). *Metu Neter, Vol. 2.* New York, NY: Khamit Corporation.

Asante, M.K. (2000). *The Egyptian Philosophers: Ancient African Voices From Imhotep to Akhenaten.* Chicago, IL: African Emerican Images.

Chang, S. (1986). *Tao of Sexology.* Reno, NV: Tao Publishing.

Holy Bible.

Kahn, H.I. (1981). *Spiritual Dimensions in Psychology.* Lebanon, NY: Omega Publishing.

Lynch, W. (1912, 1999). *The Making of a Slave.* Vensenville, IL: Lushena Books.

Maharaj, N. (1973). *I AM THAT.* Bombay, India: Chetana Publishing.

Ming-Dao, D. (1992). *365 Tao: Daily Meditations.* New York, NY: HarperCollins Publishers.

Morrow, A. (2003). *Breaking the Curse of Willie Lynch.* St. Louis, MO: Rising Sun Publications.

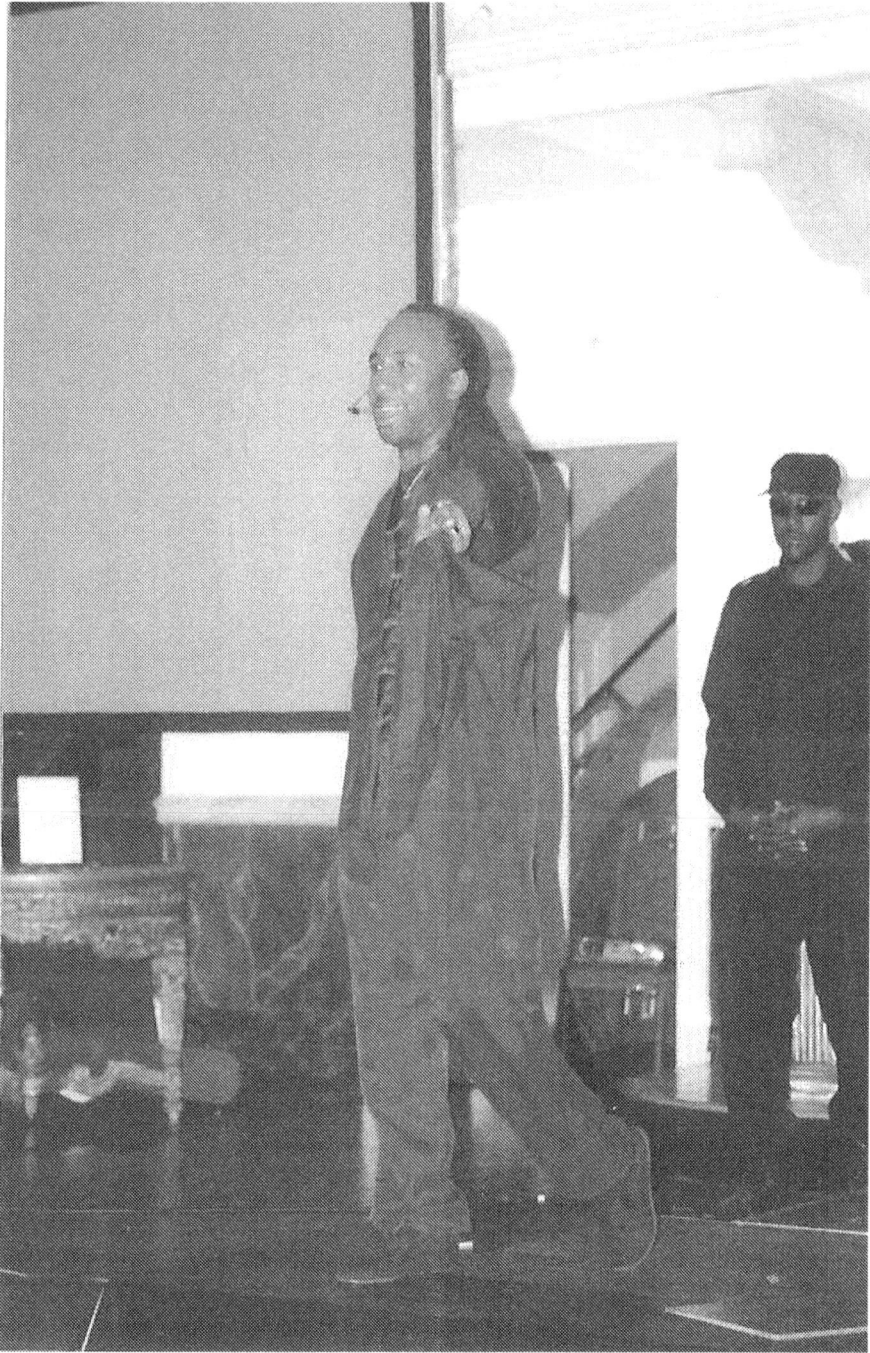

Art & Artists

Tribute To The Black Woman, is the complementary follow-up to the *Tribute to the Black Woman* CD which was released in 2003 by St. Louis native M.P.E.R.O.R.

Motivated by the notions that most artists lack self-respect and no nation can rise higher than its woman, he released the CD and subsequent **Tribute To The Black Woman** book in hopes of erasing the internal sadness resulting from the apparent adjustment Black women are making to being degraded by a number of the popular Black male Hip-Hop artists.

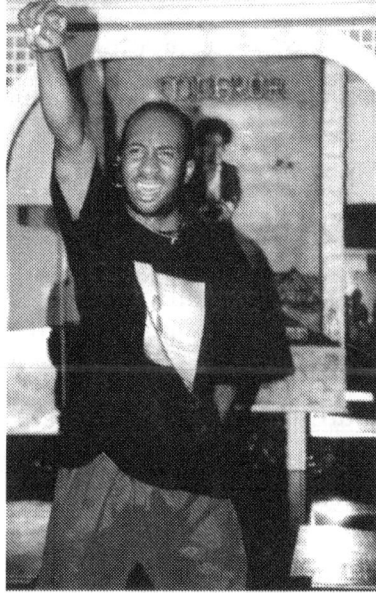

M.P.E.R.O.R. (Most Powerful Entering Resurrection Outside Ra) has had his powerful rap music heard on the radio, but felt that was not enough to properly pay homage to the power sustaining the world's people. His hope is that this book will not only provide an increased understanding, but also an overstanding of what inspired each song on the *Tribute To The Black Woman* CD.

Tribute To The Black Woman was the fourth CD released by M.P.E.R.O.R. His first was the self-titled *M.P.E.R.O.R.* released in 1996, followed by *The Rebirth* in 1999. His third CD was a collaboration with the group called T.R.U.T.H.

Squad (Transcending Righteousness Under The Heavens) on the CD *Truth or Consequences* in 2001. The fifth and most recent project is *M.P.E.R.O.R.'s Blessings*. Released in 2006, this mixed CD has three original songs, with a video shot for the song "Victory Is Mine."

Rooted in spirituality, he's no copy cat and his style is one that needs no outside validation. After all, he did prepare for 10 years before releasing his first CD. To M.P.E.R.O.R., rap is a vehicle to reach millions to change the life of at least one for the better. *mperor.com*

Kevin Bryant of Inkosi Design Studio, a St. Louis-based advertising agency, is one of several graphic artists, illustrators and photographers on staff to assist artists and entities including Nelly, Anheuser-Busch and Hallmark. *inkosidesigns.com*

Mylia Tiye Mal Jaza is a Texippian and the author of Scientific Evidence God Exists. A Fort Worth resident, the Mississippi native is also the author of six other works: Life Is Beautiful: La Vita E Bella; Life Is Beautiful: La Vita Es Hermosa; Seen In Other Words; Plea For Peace; All For Show: Film & Television Scripts; and The Old Negro and The New Negro by T. LeRoy Jefferson, M.D. *myliajaza.gq.nu*

Mari "Mary" Jefferson is a journalist, editor, vocalist, public speaker, model, business consultant, voice-over artist, publicist, visual expressionist, technical writer, and owner of several ventures in Dallas/Fort Worth including The Conglomerate, ARTiculation, The Writers Consortium and BePublished – which helps artists publish books and CDs. *bepublished.org*

ISBN: 978-0-6151-6332-1

www.ingramcontent.com/pod-product-compliance
Lightning Source LLC
Chambersburg PA
CBHW031215270326
41931CB00006B/564